Your Smear Test

Your Smear Test

A guide to screening, colposcopy and the prevention of cervical cancer

GRAHAM H. BARKER, FRCS, MRCOG

Illustrations by Jennie Smith

Adamson Books
London

Text copyright © 1987 Graham H. Barker
Illustrations copyright © 1987 Adamson Books

Published by Adamson Books
6 Foxbourne Road
London SW17 8EW

Cover design by Simon Bell
Book design by Nicky Adamson

British Library Cataloguing in Publication Data
  Your smear test: a guide to screening,
  colposcopy and the prevention of
  cervical cancer.
  1. Cervix uteri—Diagnosis   2. Diagnosis
  Cytologic
  1. Title
  618.1'4   RC280.U8

ISBN 0–948543–30–2

All rights reserved. No part of this publication may be
reproduced, stored in a retrieval system, or
transmitted, in any form or by any means, electronic,
mechanical, photocopying, recording or otherwise, without
the prior permission of the publishers. Such
permission, if granted, is subject to a fee
depending on the nature of the use.

Printed in Great Britain by the Hollen Street Press

Contents

Introduction 6
1 The cervix 9
2 Having a cervical smear 17
3 Colposcopy 36
4 Local treatments 52
5 Cone biopsy 65
6 Cervical cancer 76
7 The causes of cervical abnormalities 91
8 Associated abnormalities 103
9 The emotional impact 107
10 The case for screening 115
Helpful organizations 126
Index 127

Introduction

In 1928 a Greek doctor, born on the island of Euboea but working in the USA, announced to a largely disbelieving medical profession that he could diagnose cancer in the pre-invasive stages by examining a scraping of cells from various parts of the body under the microscope. Work he had done by taking cells from the abnormal and normal uterine cervix, with the help of his wife, and applying his special stain, has now become the means of screening for those women who will develop cancer of the cervix in later life. This man – George Nicholaus Papanicolaou (1883–1962) – has not only given his name to the 'Pap' smear but has saved thousands upon thousands of women from developing cancer of the cervix.

Until screening with cervical 'Pap' smears was introduced, a woman was left to develop cervical cancer and experience symptoms such as a blood-stained vaginal discharge or postcoital bleeding which would eventually take her to a gynaecological surgeon. Her survival largely depended upon how far her cancer had spread. With cervical smear screening, pre-malignant cancer cells can be detected years before invasion and spread has taken place, and simple, effective treatment can be given in time to prevent invasion.

Currently over 2,000 women die in England and Wales each year from cervical cancer – most of these deaths are preventable.

In the last five years there has been a massive increase in

pre-invasive cervical cancers, which have now reached epidemic proportions. But we have the means of detecting and treating cervical cancer in its early pre-invasive stage and the opportunity of drastically reducing the number of women who die from cervical cancer. The success of our screening programme depends upon the provision of adequate facilities to take, record and report on cervical smears, upon the regular invitation of women at risk to attend for a cervical smear, upon adequate facilities to evaluate and treat women with abnormal smears, and upon the willingness of all women to come forward for screening.

Nearly four million cervical smears are currently taken in Britain every year. Some of them will be reported as showing severe abnormalities which may progress to cancer, or mild abnormalities which may resolve, or may reveal infections, and some will not have sufficient cells for confident analysis. All of the women from whom this wide variety of smears has been taken will be told that their smear report is not 'negative'; all of these women will be concerned to know why and will want an explanation of the reasons and the implications. Many of them will be asked to have an examination in a colposcopy clinic. What happens there? Some will be told they need treatment for pre-cancerous conditions. What are these treatments and what do they involve?

What are the causes of abnormal smears? What are the influences of sexual behaviour on the development of cervical cancer? Why is it that in some countries the number of women who die each year from cervical cancer is falling already? Why is Britain not among them?

The answers to all these questions are becoming clearer. The last decade has seen tremendous advances in the understanding and prevention of cervical cancer and there is much information and explanation that can be given to women at risk. Unfortunately, such counselling is not always easy to obtain. Firstly, women who have just received the news of an abnormal smear are upset and may not be able to take in a great deal of information in a busy clinic or GP surgery. Secondly, many of the health care workers involved in the screening programme – i.e., receptionists, clerks, nurses, practice managers and even some doctors – may not be in a position to answer some or all of the questions women with an abnormal smear may pose. Thirdly, many clinicians actively involved in this work do not have the time available that they would like in order to counsel each woman fully, whether it be concerning a simple infection detected on the smear or a severe abnormality requiring urgent evaluation in a colposcopy clinic.

This book was written to explain in depth the whole process – from the taking of the cervical smear through reporting, colposcopy and treatment. There is also a section on the treatment of invasive cervical cancer. The text, I hope, will provide a thorough explanation for women who are about to have a cervical smear taken, for those who have unanswered questions about smear results, and for those who face the prospect of a colposcopy examination and treatment. I also hope it will be of interest to those nurses, receptionists, clerks, administrators and teachers working in this area of health care.

My great desire to produce such a book as this was fortunately reciprocated by Nicky and Stephen Adamson, of Adamson Books, who readily combined their continuing personal interest in making health care understandable with their extensive editorial and publishing expertise and experience. To Jennie Smith, whose sympathetic illustrations have greatly enhanced this book throughout, I also wish to express my gratitude, and to Shelley Power of Inpra for keeping me in order, and to my wife, Esther, for her help and thoughtful suggestions.

Graham H. Barker,
London, 1987

1 The cervix

The cervix, or neck of the womb, is a more complex organ than you may have first thought. In order to understand how pre-cancerous abnormalities can develop in its tissues and how they can be treated, it is important to have some idea of the structure and function of the cervix, and to have all the medical and technical terms associated with it explained. You will find these terms referred to again and again throughout this book, and during consultations if you require treatment following a positive smear test. Rather than repeating the definitions every time they are mentioned, almost all the terms you are likely to come across are defined in some detail in this chapter.

It's worth bearing in mind that when you have a smear test, a small number of cells are scraped off the surface of your cervix – they are so small that they have to be examined by a skilled laboratory technician under a microscope, who, as you will see in Chapter 2, will be looking for subtle but significant changes to individual cells or even parts of cells. So it is not simply the overall structure of the cervix that has to be explained, but also the make-up of individual cells, because it is here that pre-cancerous changes first take place.

Where is the cervix?

Often referred to as the neck of the womb, the cervix is the lower part of the uterus (womb) which is situated at the top of the vagina. The rest of the uterus protrudes into the abdominal cavity behind the bladder, with the rectum (the lower part of the large bowel connected to the anus) behind it. About 80 per cent of uteruses point forward (this is called anteversion), and about 20 per cent point backwards (this is called retroversion). If your womb is retroverted, your cervix points straight down the vagina; when it is anteverted, your cervix may be angled more towards the back, of the top of the vagina.

Size and structure

The cervix is on average about 2–3cm (1–1½in.) across, but its size varies considerably from woman to woman. It often enlarges after childbirth. It has a hole filled with mucus through its centre, which connects it to the cavity inside the uterus. This mucus becomes flowing and abundant the time of ovulation in the middle of your menstrual cycle (the time when you are most likely to become pregnant), but after the menopause (change of life), at around 50 years of age, the cervical mucus tends to dry up.

The central hole in the cervix allows menstrual fluid to escape from the uterine cavity during your period and, after sexual intercourse, allows sperm to enter the uterus and travel up to the Fallopian tubes to fertilize the ovum that is released each month by your ovary. Cervical mucus is very important to sperm as it washes them free of certain proteins. Without this 'washing' (a process called capacitation), sperm would be unable to break into the ovum to fertilize it.

The appearance of the cervix is very much like the top of a polished button mushroom with a hole. If you use a diaphragm (cap) for contraceptive purposes or have an intra-uterine contraceptive device fitted (a coil or IUD) you will probably be used to feeling your own cervix, as a diaphragm has to fit over and round the cervix, and you will probably have been shown how to feel if the strings of your IUD are protruding from the cervix. In this case you

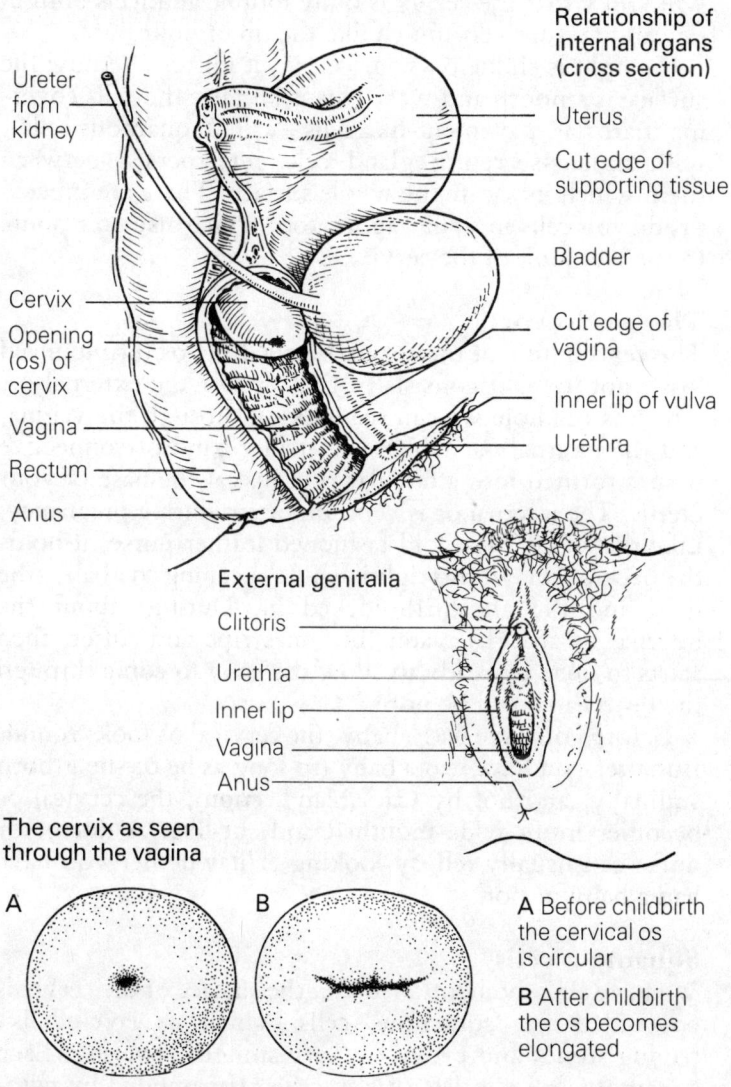

The relationship of the cervix to the other organs around it. The bladder is in front of the cervix, the ureters from the kidneys pass on either side and the large bowel (rectum) is behind.

will know that the cervix is quite mobile and feels both in size and texture very much like the tip of your nose.

If a light is shone on your cervix, it glistens because the surface is smooth and wet. This is because the cells covering it are flat, pavement-like cells – called squamous cells – with mucus-secreting gland cells interspersed between them which lubricate the whole surface. There are mucus-producing cells in your vagina, too, which also contribute to the wet look of the cervix.

The cervical os
The central hole of the cervix is called the os (pronounced 'oss', not 'oz'). It consists of two parts – the external os, which is the hole we can see looking through the vagina, and the internal os, which is a strong band of connective tissues formed into a circular ring just at the base of your uterus. The internal os is very important during pregnancy. Like the string of an old fashioned leather purse, it holds the neck of the womb tightly shut – keeping the baby, the fluid and the afterbirth locked in. During labour the internal os absorbs water, becomes ripe and softer, then starts to open up ready to allow the baby to come through the birth canal and be born.

Before you have had a baby, the cervical os looks round. But after you have had a baby (so long as he or she is born vaginally, and not by Caesarean section), the cervical os becomes more wide-mouthed and slit-like. A doctor or nurse can usually tell by looking at it whether you have had a baby or not.

Squamous cells
We have already mentioned that the surface of the cervix is covered in flat 'squamous' cells, which are layered like paving stones and provide a very smooth covering. Each squamous cell consists of a nucleus, surrounded by cytoplasm. The surface top layer is referred to as the squamous epithelium. At the base of the squamous cell layer is a very important structure called the basement membrane – more of this later.

THE CERVIX

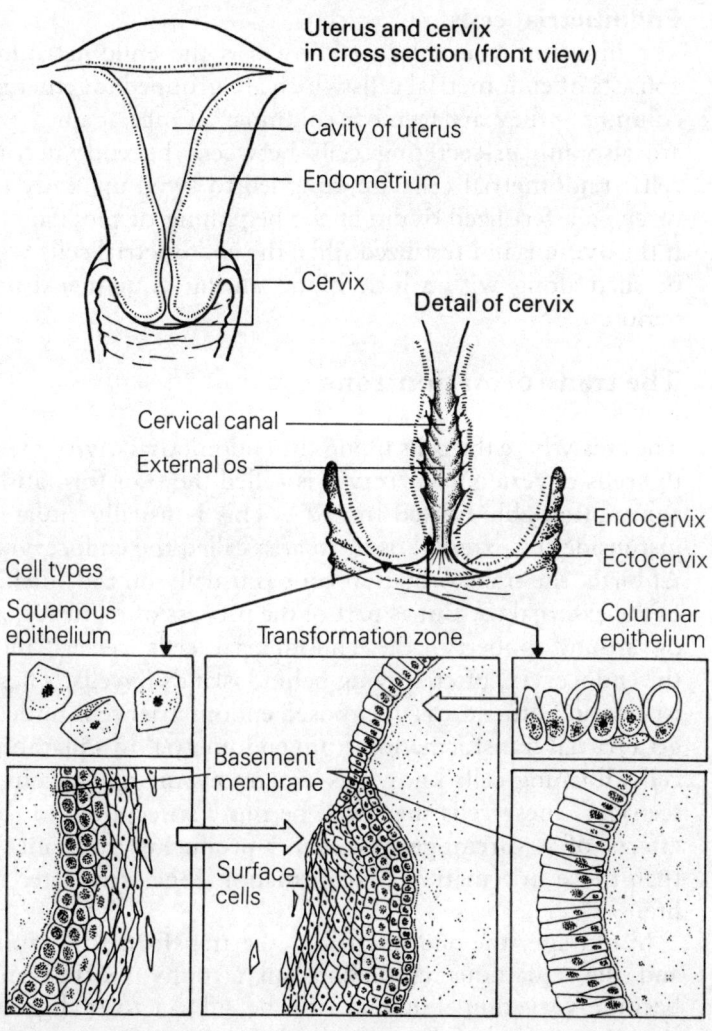

The part of the cervix most likely to undergo cancerous changes is the junction between the columnar cells of the endometrium and the squamous cells of the cervix – the transformation zone. It is from this area that cells will be taken during a cervical smear test. In some women this junction is clearly visible, in others it is hidden higher up in the cervical canal.

Endometrial cells

The lining of your uterus (known as the endometrium) consists of endometrial cells which are grouped together in columns – they are termed 'columnar'. Once again there are also mucus-secreting cells between the endometrial cells. Endometrial cells are designed to swell up ready to received a fertilized ovum at the beginning of pregnancy. If the ovum is not fertilized, then the endometrial cells will be shed along with a little blood during your menstrual period.

The transformation zone

The area where the cells lining the endometrial cavity meet the cells covering your cervix is called the transformation zone, often abbreviated to 'TZ'. This is usually situated just inside the external os in an area called the endocervix. At birth, the transformation zone is usually on the outside of the external os. But as part of the process of maturity, at or around puberty, the endometrial cells retreat into the endocervix, often leaving behind islands of cells. These islands and other areas of exposed endometrial cells undergo a partial transformation from endometrial to squamous cells, forming cells known as 'squamous metaplasia'. In a teenager, these cells may well be more susceptible to the effects of a carcinogen (a cancer-producing substance), than those in a mature transformation zone, seen later in life.

In old age, the endometrium, the transformation zone and the squamous epithelium all atrophy (wither and become very thin) but may still be subject to malignant changes, probably following initial changes which happened many years earlier but lay dormant. However, it is in the transformation zone – where the endometrial cells meet the squamous cells – that cancers of the cervix usually begin, and it is the cells of the transformation zone (at the squamo-columnar junction) which must be checked when you have a cervical smear.

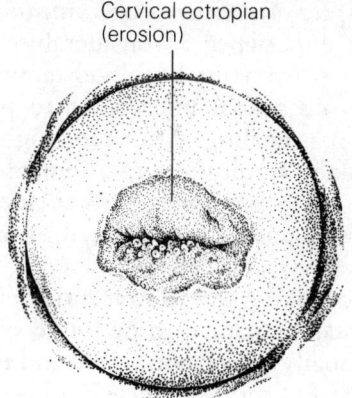

Cervical ectropian (erosion)

In an ectropian, the columnar cells lining the uterus appear on the surface of the cervix.

'Cervical erosion'

Sometimes the transformation zone may spread over a considerable area of the cervix. The correct name for this is 'cervical ectropian', but because the exposed endometrial cells appear red and velvety, they were once thought to look like an ulcer – hence the misleading but widespread term, 'cervical erosion'.

Large ectropians can occur spontaneously. They usually do not produce any symptoms, and providing that your cervical smear is negative, they don't need any treatment. Some large ectropians produce excessive quantities of mucus discharge which may be heavy enough to cause you to wear a sanitary pad. Often the damp vagina and vulva become irritated by this constant discharge and you may think you have 'thrush'. However 'thrush' is something different – it is a yeast infection of the cervix and vagina which also causes irritation (see Chapter 2). Many women are however mis-diagnosed as having 'thrush' and given anti-fungal pessaries to clear it, when in fact they have an ectropian, so the discharge continues.

If you have an ectropian which is causing symptoms like these, your doctor will probably refer you to a gynaecological clinic for treatment by some form of cautery, either with a freezing probe (cryocautery – see Chapter 4), which does not require general anaesthetic, or a hot wire cautery (see Chapter 4) which does. Immediately after cautery you may experience a considerable mucus discharge which may occasionally be bloodstained, and you'll be advised to avoid sexual intercourse to prevent infection while the cervix is healing. After a fortnight or so new squamous cells usually cover the area occupied by the ectropian and a new transformation zone is formed – in the more normal position within the external os and the endocervix.

If you are pregnant, or taking the contraceptive pill, it is quite common for a small ectropian to be found on your cervix. These do not usually cause symptoms and may be left alone, providing a recent cervical smear has been taken and is found to be negative.

Nabothian follicles
Sometimes one or more small, clear fluid-filled cysts may be found on the cervix. These are called Nabothian follicles and occur because occasionally the mucus ducts in the cervical surface get blocked and then swell up with mucoid fluid. They do not usually produce any symptoms and do not require any treatment. To the naked eye their appearance is similar to that of small grapes. Biblical scholars like to point out that in the Bible Naboth had a vineyard (I Kings xxi), and that this must be the origin of the term 'Nabothian' follicles. In fact, the reason for the name is more prosaic. The follicles were first described by Martin Naboth (1675-1721), a German Professor of Medicine in Leipzig. He may well have drunk wine, but there is no record of him having had a vineyard!

2 Having a smear test

The cervical smear test is designed to identify pre-cancerous abnormalties in the cells of the cervix so that treatment can be given in good time to prevent cancer developing. What actually causes the abnormality in the first place is still not entirely clear, although contributing factors are known. What is clear, however, is that if these abnormalities are caught early enough, they can be completely eradicated, and the smear test is the first step in this process. It is an incredibly simple, painless procedure, which takes a few seconds. No matter what your age or background, if you are or have been sexually active, it is a good idea to have regular tests done, as they can save your life.

Unlike many other forms of cancer, cervical cancer can be detected and successfully treated very early. In those countries where women are personally invited to attend for regular screening with cervical smears it has been clearly demonstrated that this is effective in reducing the chances of dying from cervical cancer. However, in the United Kingdom and many other countries there is no co-ordinated national screening system, and it is left to individual women to get access to regular screening as best they can.

Where to go varies, and you will have to approach your general practitioner, family planning clinic, well woman clinic or woman screening clinic. The availability of the facilities is different in different parts of the country, and you may have to go to some trouble to make the arrangements. How often the tests are performed will also vary, although regular screening is essential – about once every three years. Moreover, recall systems, to invite women back for a further test after the necessary interval, are still unusual. Hopefully, they will become widely operational and will bring in women who would otherwise be left out.

But for the time being, it is up to each woman to ensure that she has appointments for smears. Everybody has a natural reluctance to delve into the medical unknown, whether it is for a dental check for a child or a blood pressure count for a businessman, for nobody wants to be told that they should wear a brace on their teeth and nobody wants to be told that they are overweight and smoke too much. However, prevention is better than cure.

Where to go

You can ask to be tested by your general practitioner (most of whom gallantly ignore the fact that they are not paid directly for taking smears from women who are under 35 years of age). Family planning clinics offer regular smear tests, as do the relatively few 'well women' clinics currently in existence. In some parts of the country early diagnostic centres have been set up, some of which are supported by charity and small donations from the women who attend. Alternatively, you can ask at your local health centre or Community Health Council office (address in the telephone book) if there is one of these in your area. If you are expecting a baby, you will also be offered a routine cervical smear at your first antenatal check-up.

The availability of smear test facilities varies throughout the country and it may be necessary for you to travel, to take time from work, to arrange a baby sitter, to telephone around, to leave no stone unturned until you get regular cervical smears. If the smear is abnormal then you will need to be seen in a colposcopy clinic – more of this later – and again the provision of these clinics around the country is patchy. General practitioners have the right to refer patients to any clinic they feel is appropriate so you may need to travel to get access to a colposcopy examination.

Until a better system is introduced, the onus is on you to check that the smear report showed no abnormalities, although some units do notify results by letter. The result of your smear will usually come direct to the antenatal clinic too, if you have one there. It is usually your responsibility to ask for further smears on a regular basis as well.

How often to be tested

How frequently smears are performed depends on several local factors. This is usually made into a local policy, which your doctor or clinic nurse will tell you about. It will often depend on the state of local laboratory facilities – many of which are extremely understaffed and overstretched. The official recommended interval between smear tests is every five years, although most experts agree that every three years is probably the minimum safe interval and individual clinics and doctors may offer more frequent smears. Some health districts have now set up computerized 'recall' systems, although they are in the minority, and the amount of money available to fund these quite complex arrangements has been insufficient for the size of the problem. Many GPs have actually set up their own 'recall' systems, often without the help of a computer.

If your doctor thinks there is some particular reason that you may be at high risk of cervical cancer, such as a family history of the disease, he or she may offer annual smear tests. You will certainly be advised to have an annual test if you ever have a positive report which requires treatment, or if you have ever been infected with a sexually transmitted disease, especially genital warts (see Chapter 7).

When to be tested

Once you have established where you can have a cervical smear taken it is best to arrange to have a cervical smear taken between menstrual periods as heavy blood staining may prevent a good view of the smear. If you are to have the test at the beginning or end of a period a small amount of bleeding may not matter, but check with the nurse or doctor beforehand.

How the smear is taken

In order to take a cervical smear the doctor or nurse must insert a vaginal speculum to separate the vaginal walls and obtain a good view of the cervix. You will be invited to lie on the examination bed either on your back with your knees drawn up and apart, or on your left side with your knees drawn up to your chest. The speculum used most frequently is the duck-billed type called after a surgeon named Edward Cusco, and originally developed in Paris in the early nineteenth century. It was designed for surgical operations, and has a little nut and bolt to hold and keep it open. However, since taking a cervical smear only takes a few seconds this function is not required.

The speculum is gently passed along the length of the vagina until it reaches the cervix. The handles are then squeezed together and the two valves of the speculum open up a short distance to reveal the cervix at the end of the vagina. If the uterus is very anteverted it sometimes takes a little manoeuvring with the end of the speculum to get the cervix into view. A good light is needed so that the doctor or nurse can see and inspect the cervix thoroughly.

Some centres use a disposable speculum made of plastic which is only used once, but most centres will use the stainless steel ones which can be sterilized and re-used.

Inspecting the cervix
With the speculum in place your cervix can be scrutinized along with the upper part of the vagina. The doctor will note any excessive discharge, and if there is any sign of infection, he will take a swab and send it to the laboratory for analysis. The surface of the cervix is inspected carefully for the presence of abnormal blood vessels (which may suggest an early cancer), an ectropian (see Chapter 1), or

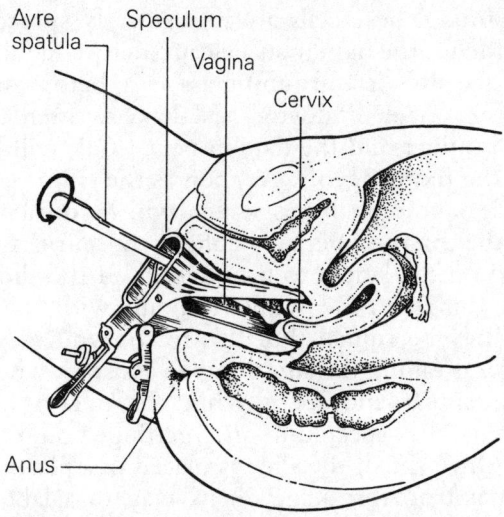

To take a cervical smear, the doctor displays the cervix using a vaginal speculum. Surface cells are removed from the cervix by rotating a special spatula two or three times against it.

warts. In women after the menopause (change of life) the appearance of the cervical surface will to a certain extent be rather thin (this is termed atrophic). This occurs as a result of the fall in oestrogen levels when the ovaries cease to produce the hormone at the menopause.

Taking the smear

A thin layer of cells is taken from the cervix and the entrance to the cervical canal using a long, specially shaped intrument called a spatula. A commonly used type is named after a Canadian from Montreal – J. Ernest Ayre – who first described it in 1947. Ayre spatulas are made of wood, rather like ice lolly sticks. They are produced by the thousands and are disposable. The spatula is passed through the speculum to your cervix and the longer end is placed in the external os. It is rotated two or three times with a little pressure to ensure a good layer of cells is obtained from the transformation zone. This procedure is not painful. These cells are immediately spread in a thin smear (hence the name) on a clean microscope slide. At the end of the slide is a ground glass area; before the smear is taken the nurse or doctor will have written on it your name, number and the date in pencil (ink will be washed off by the fixing agent). As soon as the smear is placed on the slide, avoiding blobs which will be difficult to view down the microscope, an alcohol-type spirit is washed or sprayed on the smear to fix the cells. If the slide is left in the air for any time without fixing with the spirit the smear may be ruined. For this reason you may find that whoever is taking the smear has an assistant who will plate out the smear and fix it while the doctor or nurse is removing the speculum and getting you comfortable again. Once fixed, the slide is placed in a plastic carrier to protect it from breakage on its way to a laboratory for analysis. The whole procedure takes about half a minute.

An additional spatula or brush
The area of the cervix which is most at risk of developing a cancer is just inside the external os – within the endocervix. Various devices have been produced to obtain more cells from that area than can presently be obtained with an Ayre spatula. In the USA, considerable attention has been given to obtaining cells from the endocervix using a tiny brush (a miniature version of the large brushes used to clean bottles such as milk bottles). Cotton wool-tipped swabs have also been taken from the upper vagina near the cervix to make sure all abnormal cells are picked up.

In the United Kingdom some units take an extra smear using a spatula with a longer point to obtain more cells from the endocervix.

The cytology form

Each microscope slide on which there is a cervical smear must be accompanied by a cytology form (the word 'cytology' means the study of cells). This documentation is usually done before the smear is taken. In the United

Kingdom there is a standard form used by many cytology laboratories which is divided into three main sections. The form contains a number of duplicates so that general practitioners and other centres can be informed of the result, to help with recall systems and to prevent duplication of smear taking and missing abnormal results.

The left side of the form includes sections for your file number, name, address, date of birth and the address of your general practitioner and other centres to be informed of the result. There is also a box for your occupation or, if you are married, the occupation of your partner. This is an antique means of helping place you in a social class. I will not go into this cumbersome classification but gathering this information has helped to track the course of cervical cancer and pre-cancers amongst various social classes. However, many of the findings of the early work done on the effects of social class on this disease are now becoming out of date and it is clear that the assumptions made about social class over the last 25 years will not hold for the next decade or so. A more relevant question on this form would be whether you smoke or not (see Chapter 7), but this is not currently asked.

The right side of the form is divided in two – the upper half contains more details about the woman plus the date of taking the smear, the date of the last smear and the date of the first day of the last menstrual period. Further clinical information is given to the cytologist such as: 'Is the woman pregnant?' (Many smears are taken at antenatal booking clinics or at clinics dealing with requests for termination of pregnancy.) Is she on the oral contraceptive pill? Is she wearing an intra-uterine contraceptive device? Has she been pregant before? There is also a little box where the doctor or nurse can give a report on the state of the cervix – 'ectropian', 'polyps' etc. – and a large box for writing out relevant clinical information.

The lower half of the right hand side of the form is the area where the cytologist reports on the smear and makes recomendations such as 'refer for coloposcopy' – more of this later.

YOUR SMEAR TEST

| 01 PATIENT'S HOSPITAL OR CLINIC CASE REFERENCE NO. | A12345 | 10 NAME AND ADDRESS (TOWN) OF LABORATORY | | 11 SLIDE SERIAL NO. | |

02
- SURNAME: SMITH MAIDEN NAME:
- FIRST NAMES: JANE
- FULL POSTAL ADDRESS:

03
- A — NAME AND ADDRESS OF SENDER: MR. CAREFUL — CONSULTANT, GYNAECOLOGY CLINIC — WARD
- IF NOT GP — IF HOSPITAL STATE: HOSPITAL
- Fold for B

04 DATE OF BIRTH — DAY 01 MONTH 04 YEAR 64
Fold for A

05 M/S NO.

06 SOURCE OF SMEAR: GP 1 AHA 2 FP CLINIC 3 HOSPITAL (4) Other 5

07 HUSBAND'S OCCUPATION (patient's if unmarried) also state if Manager, Foreman or other: MEDIA SALES

08
- B — NAME AND ADDRESS OF GP: DR. FRIENDLY, THE HEALTH CENTRE

09 SPECIMEN TYPE: Cervical scrape (1) Vaginal sample 2 Cyto pipette 4 Other (specify) 8   LOCAL CODES 26 27 28 29 30

Request/Report/Recall Form for Cervical or Vaginal Cytology – LAB's COPY

---

12 MARITAL STATE: Single (1) Married 2 Widowed 3 Divorced 3

13 PREGNANCIES:
- Total births (live and still): 0
- Total of abortions and miscarriages: 0

14 CONDITION: Pregnant 1 Post-natal (under 12 weeks) 2 IUCD fitted 16 On oral contraceptive 4 On other hormones (specify in Box 21) 8

15 DATE OF THIS TEST: DAY 01 MTH 6 YR 87
16 LMP (1st day): 15 / 05 / 87
17 LAST TEST: / / 84
18 NO PREVIOUS TEST (put x)

19 SYMPTOMS:
- Discharge 1
- Post-coital bleeding (2)
- Inter-menstrual bleeding 4
- Post-menopausal bleeding 8
- Other symptoms 16 (Specify in Box 21)

20 APPEARANCE OF CERVIX: Normal 1 Eroded (2) Cervicitis 4 Polyps 8 Malignant 16

21 CLINICAL DATA (PREVIOUS TREATMENT INCLUDING RADIO THERAPY/CHEMOTHERAPY)

Post-coital bleeding

signature V. Careful

22 CYTOLOGY REPORT

Candida albicans seen
Sheets of cells showing
severe dysplasia

23 EVIDENCE OF NEOPLASIA CYTOLOGICAL PATTERN SUGGESTS:
- Inadequate specimen 1
- Negative 2
- Mild dysplasia 3
- Severe dysplasia/carcinoma-in-situ (4)
- Carcinoma-in-situ/? invasive 5
- ? Glandular neoplasia 6

24 INFLAMMATION: Severe Inflammatory Change 1 Trichomonas 2 Candida (4) Viral 8

25 FURTHER INVESTIGATION SUGGESTED: Repeat smear in ___ months 1 or after treatment 2 Colposcopy (16) Cervical biopsy 4 Uterine curettage 8

Signature F. Punctilious date 25.6.87

The cytology laboratory

In the United Kingdom many cytology laboratories – where smears are analyzed – are currently overloaded with backlogs of unreported slides, so the report may be made and sent back to the doctor or nurse in two days or two or more months – depending on the state of the laboratory work load. Cytologists are highly trained and there are not enough of them at the moment. Each slide must be individually examined by a cytologist as there are no means, as yet, of examining these slides with machines, although people are working on the idea.

In the cytology laboratory your cervical smear will be stained, using Papanicolaou's stain. This stains the cells so that the nuclei in the centre appear blue and the fluid surrounding the nuclei (the cytoplasm) greeny orange.

The smear is then scrutinized under the microscope. If it looks normal it wll be reported on the form as 'negative' and a ring placed round number two on the smear form. If there are not enough cells present on the slide to be sure that all is normal the report will be 'inadequate specimen', that is, insufficient for complete reassurance, and a ring placed round number one on the smear form. If the specimen was inadequate, the cytologist may recommend that the smear is repeated after a time interval of two or three months, when the cells on the cervix will have regenerated.

Copies of the report are sent to the doctor or nurse who took the smear (with a copy to your general practitioner if necessary) and if it was inadequate you will receive a letter asking you to return for a repeat smear. This often causes alarm and you might assume that something awful has been discovered, when in fact a repeat smear is only required because the cytologist cannot see enough cells to be happy to write 'negative'.

Opposite: An example of the cytology form which accompanies your smear to the laboratory. Boxes 22 to 25 show an example of a 'positive' report which needs urgent action.

Inflammatory smears

Occasionally the squamous cells from the cervix are completely or almost completely obscured on the slide by the presence of large numbers of white blood cells (pus cells); the cytologist will report 'inflammatory smear – please repeat after treatment'. Sometimes the cervical cells are obscured by large numbers of bacteria (often cocci) and the cytologist will report 'coccal haze' and again ask for a repeat smear after treatment.

Occasionally a large cervical ectropian may become mildly infected (so-called cervicitis) and this will require treatment before a clear smear can be reported with confidence. Again this can cause unnecessary alarm if you received a letter to ask you to make an appointment for a repeat smear because the report was 'inflammatory'.

If your smear report indicates this type of inflammatory infection, your doctor may suggest that he or she takes a high vaginal swab (which simply means taking a sample of the fluids high up on the vaginal walls) which will be sent to the laboratory for microbiological culture. The laboratory will then send back a report on what type of microorganism is causing the infection and the doctor can prescribe a suitable antibiotic medicine to clear it up. Other doctors may simply prefer to prescribe a 'blanket' antibiotic – one that is known to cure several different types of infection – without going through the process of taking a swab.

Specific infections

Some specific infections which are nothing whatever to do with cancer can be identified from a smear and the cytologist will indicate them on the form where necessary. If one of these infections is found, the doctor or nurse who took the smear will direct you to the right treatment through your GP. Finding these infections is an added benefit of the smear test which is not widely known.

Thrush

Thrush is an infection of the vagina and cervix (often involving the vulva) which leaves yellowy-white creamy blobs over the vaginal surface; these are said to resemble the flecked appearance of a thrush's breast feathers, hence the name. It is not a marked resemblance actually, and the word frequently causes confusion. One lady told me that she had recently recovered from a nasty dose of 'thrust' – well, perhaps she had. The organism causing thrush is a yeast which has two common names – candida (candida albicans) and monilia. Sometimes the condition is referred to as candidiasis or moniliasis – but 'thrush' is the popular alternative name.

It may cause vaginal and vulval irritation, leading to pain during intercourse.

The strands of monilia as they appear under the microscope can be easily identified by the cytologist viewing the cervical smear. It is usually treated by giving pessaries to insert into the vagina – either a one- or three-day treatment, which have largely superseded the cheaper fourteen day treatment using nystatin (so called because it was discovered in New York State).

Many women may experience pain and itching in the vulva or vagina, describing it as 'thrush' even though it is not caused by a monilia infection. For instance, tight trousers or synthetic fibre underwear may produce vulval irritation in some women which is not always due to monilia (especially if it develops in a few minutes or hours). Another myth is that thrush is more common in women who take the oral contraceptive pill – extensive research has shown that thrush is no more common in 'pill' users than it is in women who use barrier methods of contraception, or in women who use no contraception at all. However, thrush is commonly seen in pregnant women.

Thrush tends to affect sexually active women, and some doctors offer treatment for the male partner in the hope of preventing cross-infection. Thrush infection of the penis is not common in men but they may pass the yeast on. However, the vagina must be susceptible before thrush will develop; this generally means that the natural bacteria which usually live in an happy colony in the vagina will have been disturbed in some way before they permit the overgrowth of the yeast. Severe illness can, of course, do this but this is rarely the explanation in the large numbers of healthy young women who are bothered by thrush.

Gardnerella

Gardnerella vaginalis is a vaginal infection from an organism called after one of its discoverers, H.L. Gardner (with C.D. Dukes). It is part of a syndrome called bacterial vaginosis. It produces a greyish mucoid discharge with a particularly unpleasant smell. Itching (doctors refer to genital itching as 'pruritis') is not as troublesome with Gardnerella discharge as it is with thrush.

The cytologist will be alerted to the presence of bacterial vaginosis on a smear test by the appearance of certain 'clue cells' – squamous cells covered by small bacilli. In fact you may find that you are offered treatment for Gardnerella infection found on your cervical smear before you develop the symptoms of the vaginal discharge.

The standard anti-yeast treatment with pessaries used against thrush is not totally effective against bacterial vaginosis and they usually need treatment with a course of metronidazole tablets. These occasionally interact with alcohol in some people, so alcoholic drinks should be avoided when the tablets are being taken.

Trichomonas

A vaginal infection with an organism called Trichomonas vaginalis often produces a bubbly discharge with a greenish tinge. However, the discharge may not always have this appearance and is sometimes mistaken for Gardnerella, or vice versa. Under the microscope there is no doubt. The trichomonad is an heart-shaped organism called a protozoon, and will move around in a blob of discharge by thrashing its whip-like flagellae. Even in the fixed cervical smear preparation the cytologist will have no difficulty in recognizing trichomonads.

The treatment of Trichomonas vaginalis infections is again a course of metronidazole tablets. Cross infection with trichomonas can be a problem and so if you are found to have this infection your doctor may offer treatment to your partner as well. Metronidazole tablets can be taken over a week or in big doses over one or two days – this latter method avoids the prolonged alcohol abstinence recommended, but occasionally causes nausea. Many doctors will offer treatment if trichomonas organisms are seen on the cervical smear even if the woman in question has not yet developed symptoms.

Gonococcus (gonorrhoea)
The signs of gonorrhoea infection – pelvic pain and a thick purulent discharge in the vagina – usually only appear after the infection has taken a severe hold. It can be picked up before symptoms develop by taking special swabs and examining them using special stains. Occasionally, the gonococcus, which causes gonorrhoea, can be detected by the cytologist from a routine cervical smear, although this may be very difficult. The Papanicolaou stain is not as good as some other microbiological stains for showing up these organisms.

The treatment is a special form of antibiotic therapy given at a clinic specializing in venereal diseases. These clinics, which used to be called Special Clinics and are now called Departments of Genito-Urinary Medicine, also operate a contact tracing service to ensure that anyone at risk can be offered treatment.

The term 'venereal disease' clinic or VD Clinic for short is seldom used now, as it isn't completely accurate. Some of the diseases for which they offer treatment are venereally – or sexually – transmitted ('venereal' comes from Venus, goddess of Love) and some are not, for instance some types of vaginal infection. These clinics offer a valuable opportunity for having a cervical smear performed as well as swabs for infection. This is particularly important for women who attend these clinics for the treatment of genital warts (see below), as a high proportion of them will have abnormal cervical smears. The association of abnormal smears and the human papilloma wart virus is discussed in Chapter 7.

Actinomycetes

The actinomycetes organism is a rarity, but it can be present when a woman has worn one of the older types of all-plastic intrauterine devices for a number of years, such as the 'Lippes Loop' or 'Saf-T-Coil'. Once the cytologist has reported the presence of actinomycetes, the doctor will invariably offer to remove the intra-uterine contraceptive device to prevent a chronic intrauterine infection, and will give a prolonged course of high dose pencillin. The presence of the copper banding on the more modern intrauterine contraceptive devices seems to deter the accumulation of actinomycetes.

Herpes genitalis

It is just possible that the cytologist will recognize infection of the cervix with the Herpes simplex virus, although confirmation of this will be required from the virology department of the Genito-Urinary Medicine Clinic. The appearance of the infected cells seen by the cytologist is one of single or multi-nucleated cells in which the nuclei look different.

Koilocytosis (genital wart virus)

The cytologist will be on the look-out for cells showing evidence of infection with the wart virus known as human papilloma virus (HPV). This condition is known as koilocytosis. These cells have slightly bigger than average nuclei surrounded by a halo, because the cytoplasm around them has become darker. The changes in the cell seen by the cytologist are not very different from those of mild dysplasia (early pre-cancerous change – see Chapter 3). Sometimes an acute HPV infection of the cervix will produce cells quite similar to mildly dysplastic ones. However, since HPV infection is now thought to be closely linked to the development of pre-cancerous change, if you are found to have koilocytosis, you will be referred for colposcopy.

Sometimes women with koilocytosis found on the cervical smear will have visible warts (the medical terms for a wart is condyloma) on the vulva, and/or the anus. However, many women with koilocytosis seen on their cervical smears will not have actual warts at the time, and may not have had visible warts in the past, but may have had HPV infection some years previously without actually knowing about it. The role of the human papilloma virus in the development of pre-cancerous and cancerous conditions of the cervix (and vulva) is very important – it is discussed fully in Chapter 7.

Finding out your test result

In the previous section we considered the two common causes for having a cervical smear repeated – firstly that there was an insufficient number of cells present on the glass microscope slide for the cytologist to be happy to give the 'all clear' and to say that the smear was 'negative'; and secondly, that there may have been an infection present. Sometimes the organisms of the infection, or the white blood 'pus' cells they cause to be present, may obscure the squamous cells of the cervix so much that the cytologist, again, cannot see enough normal squamous cells to be certain that all is well.

In any of the above cases the nurse or doctor who took the smear will call you back to the clinic or surgery for a repeat smear, or offer treatment for the infection before repeating the smear.

Confidentiality

Usually nurses, doctors or their secretaries and receptionists will not discuss the cytology report findings over the telephone if they are anything but completely negative – after all anyone could ring up, pretending to be the patient. Many members of staff will be happy to reply to a telephone enquiry from the woman that all is negative.

However, if the report is 'insufficient for analysis', or indicates that there is some infection present, the clinic or surgery will usually send you a written note asking you to make another appointment soon. The receipt of such a letter may be extremely alarming and you may be tempted to telephone the clinic or surgery immediately for a further explanation. However, as I have said, a further explanation will not be forthcoming, since this may be highly confidential information, especially if it concerns an infection, and the clinic nurse or receptionist has no means of verifying who a telephone enquirer may be. Also a clinic receptionist might not be able to explain what 'Gardnerella' or 'koilocytosis' might be – it is not her job – and that sort of discussion is best left for the doctor at the next appointment.

This often causes more panic and, not infrequently frustration and anger. But on reflection, I am sure that you would prefer to know that your medical affairs are not openly discussed by the clinic or surgery staff, and that your privacy and confidentiality are being both protected and respected.

The best that can be offered is a quick appointment to discuss with the doctor the findings of the smear report. Often this is mention of a trivial infection and not the bad tidings of a cancer. The previous section catalogues the variety of infections which can be indicated by the cytologist. These should be explained by your doctor to you in person, and not sent in a letter (which might conceivably be opened by someone other than yourself), or given over the telephone by unqualified staff.

If your smear is positive

Squamous cells on the surface of the cervix take some time to pass from normality to developing into a tumour cell. For many women this process may take several years – for a few women it can, unfortunately, take a matter of months. The idea of the cervical smear is to catch the cells when they are in an abnormal form, but before a cancer has developed. At this point the abnormal areas of cells can be eliminated in good time.

The cytologist looking at the cervical smear can identify changes in the squamous cells which, in a high proportion of women, would progress in later life to become a cancer. The terms applied to these cell changes are dysplasia, dyskariosis and, occasionally, atypia. The prefix 'dys' means 'bad' or 'difficult' – so dysplasia would indicate bad moulding, and dyskariosis means literally, bad nucleus. Atypia, of course, implies a change from the normal.

There are three grades of abnormality between a normal cell and a tumour cell which the cytologist can recognize – mild dysplasia, moderate dysplasia, severe dysplasia.

Mild and moderate dysplasia

There are many subtle changes which the cytologist will look for when deciding if a squamous cell is becoming dysplastic, or abnormal, but in particular there is a decrease in overall cell size, an increase in the size of the nucleus, and also a change in its appearance. The shape of the cell tends to change to a more rounded or oval form and there are significant changes in the colour of the stained cytoplasm. Mild or moderate dysplasia is usually registered on the smear report as class number 3.

Without treatment, mild dysplasia usually progresses to moderate and then severe dysplasia. However, in a smaller and unfortunately decreasing proportion of women, the mild dysplasia cells may settle down to normal after a few months, especially if they are due to inflammation from an acute viral infection such as HPV (genital warts). Many doctors now feel that women with mild dysplasia should be sent immediately for colposcopy (see Chapter 3). Other doctors prefer to to repeat the cervical smear in four to six months' time to see if the mild dysplasia has settled down.

If koilocytosis (infection with the genital wart virus) is found, then you would definitely be referred to a colposcopy clinic since a recent study showed that nearly one quarter of women with koilocytosis may also have an area of severe dysplasia when examined with a colposcope.

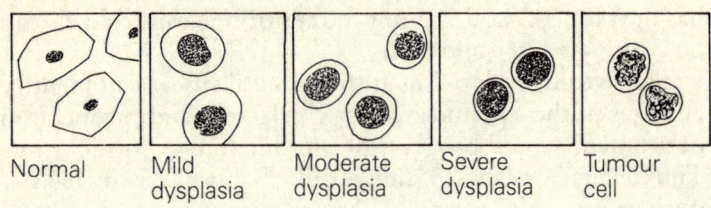

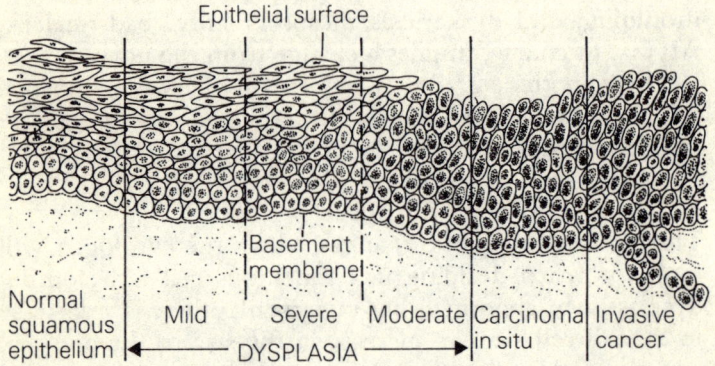

Above: The surface changes on the cervix, from normality through dysplasia to an invasive cancer. Top: Changes to the cell nuclei in a similar progression.

Severe dysplasia

Cells from the cervix showing severe dysplasia are those in which the changes described for mild dysplasia are more marked but not severe enough to be classed as an actual cancer cell – or, as it is known medically, a carcinoma cell.

The cervical smear report will usually be number 4, which also includes 'carcinoma in situ' (see below). If severe dysplasia is found on your smear you will be referred to the colposcopy clinic as soon as possible. It is now known that all but a small proportion (only around 5 per cent) of women with severe dysplasia will progress to an invasive cancer. This may take several years or only six to twelve months – so early treatment is essential as nobody can tell whether the progression to an invasive cancer will be fast or slow.

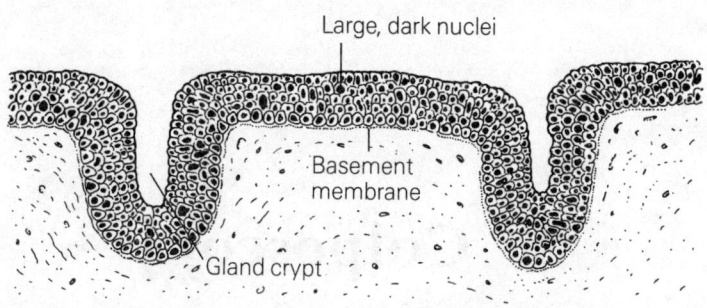

Surface cells may be found deeper in the cervix when they occur at the base of gland crypts.

Cells showing severe dysplasia usually, but not always, come from an area of the squamous epithelium on the cervical surface which consists almost completely of abnormal cells.

'Carcinoma in situ'

'Carcinoma in situ' means that actual cancer cells are found from the surface of the epithelium down to the basement membrane – but these cells have not yet penetrated through the crucial barrier of the basement membrane. In other words, there is no invasive cancer yet.

These cells are quite different from normal squamous cells. The average size of a carcinoma in situ cell is approximately one quarter that of normal, while the nucleus is about three times the size. In invasive cancer the cells are about one fifth the size of normal and their nuclei are about two to three times the size of normal cells. In carcinoma in situ (full thickness layer of abnormal cells) the cells appear on the smear singly and not often in clumps. In invasive cancer the tumour cells have a greater tendency to clump together.

In any of these situations you would be referred to a colposcopy clinic as quickly as possible to find out just what is going on.

3 Colposcopy

If your smear report discovers abnormal cells you will probably be referred to a colposcopy clinic. Referral is automatic if your smear is severely abnormal or indicates 'carcinoma in situ', and sometimes you will be referred even if the abnormality is mild or moderate, because your doctor wants you to be examined at once, to be on the safe side.

The colposcopy clinic is organized by a gynaecological oncologist – a doctor who specializes in cancers of the female reproductive organs – or by a general gynaecologist with a special interest in colposcopy work. Most colposcopy clinics are situated in teaching hospitals or district general hospitals.

What is the colposcope?

The colposcope is a binocular microscope with a field of vision which allows the whole cervix to be viewed in considerable detail, although the magnification is quite low, usually about ten times life size. The word is derived from the Greek word 'colpos', which means bay or vagina, because it is a microscope for looking through the vagina at the cervix. It can also be used for inspecting the vulva, vagina and anus for warts, or even areas of pre-cancerous abnormality on the vulva and vagina.

It was used initially in Germany in the 1920s but achieved more widespread use in Britain, the rest of Europe, USA

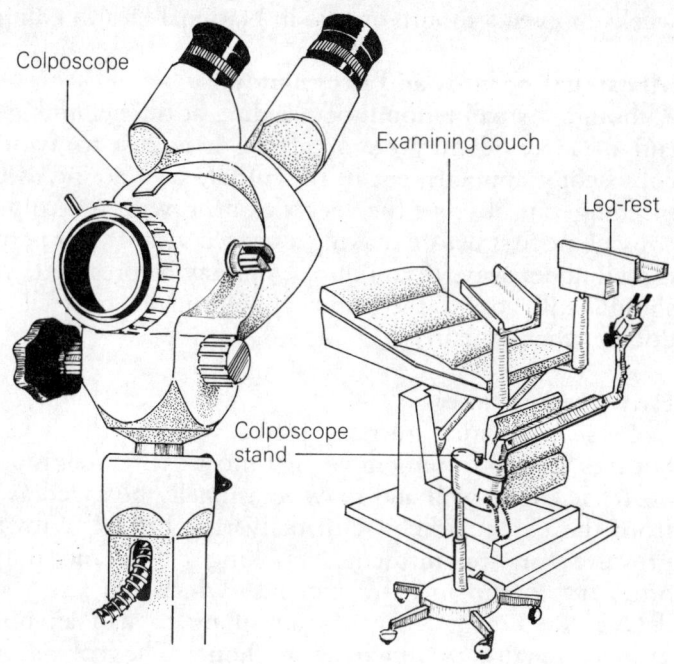

The colposcope (left) shown in detail, and in front of a specially designed examination couch (right).

and Australia in the 1960s and 1970s. Many colposcopes have side arms for teaching and taking still photographs and some are connected to a video so that the patient and student doctors can see what is happening at the same time. A basic colposcope, depending upon its quality, costs up to £10,000.

What happens at the colposcopy clinic

Your appointment for the colposcopy clinic may be several weeks from the time the abnormal cytology report of the cervical smear was issued. Urgent appointments are given for severe dysplasias and other class 4 smears, but the moderate and mild dysplasias may have to wait several weeks or even a month or two in National Health Clinics.

Menstrual periods and pregnancy

Although a small amount of bleeding at the beginning or end of a period may not interfere, it is best to avoid a colposcopy appointment in the middle of a period as the bleeding can obscure the cervix. Check with the colposcopy clinic first before making a wasted visit if your period is well under way. If you think you may be pregnant, you should still attend the clinic appointment, but tell the doctor when you arrive.

How long it takes

Colposcopy clinics are busy places. Waiting times vary, but it is as well to remember that most gynaecologists are obstetricians as well and may occasionally be called away from the clinic to help with delivering babies. With the pressure for appointments, booking clerks and nurses often try to slip in extra patients, which can also cause delays. Be prepared for a wait of up to half an hour, or occasionally as much as an hour. The colposcopic examination may take from four to eight minutes, with up to twenty minutes devoted to counselling and questioning between you and the doctor.

Initial questions

On arrival at the colposcopy clinic considerable attention will be paid to monitoring and registering you, for accurate records are absolutely essential for colposcopy work. Special colposcopy record cards are completed in addition to ordinary hospital notes, so that if the hospital notes go astray (not an unheard of occurrence!), the colposcopy details will still be available separately in the colposcopy clinic. These details will include your full address so that you can easily be contacted, and the name and address of your general practitioner, who will be kept informed of progress and treatment. Many colposcopy clinics will be doing much needed research on various aspects of cervical smear work and may ask a dozen or so questions before the examination. Many of these concern your menstrual periods – particularly the date of the first day of your last period (and any possibility of pregnancy will be checked out). Other questions cover the sort of information included on the smear form, that is, date of birth, type of contraception used, pregnancy (if any) and previous problems with cervical smears (if any). There will often be questions about occupation (for social class purposes) and whether you smoke or not, and, if so, how many each day. There may be questions about the age of first sexual intercourse and the number of sexual partners. Many of these questions may have a bearing on whether you are likely to be more at risk of cervical cancer (see Chapter 7).

Nowadays there is usually considerable interest shown in a past history of genital warts in yourself and/or your partner. Relevant symptoms, such as vaginal discharge, bleeding after sexual intercourse (post-coital bleeding, PCB), intermenstrual bleeding (IMB) or bleeding after the periods have stopped at the menopause (post-menopausal bleeding, PMB) will also be recorded in some detail.

It is particularly helpful if you can work out the date of the first day of your last menstrual period before going into the colposcopy clinic, as this question can often fox an unprepared patient and waste much valuable time while the answer is searched for.

The examination

When you enter the examination room, a nurse will invite you to lie comfortably on the couch. Many clinics have purpose-built hydraulic couches which work in a similar way to dentists' chairs, so that the height can be adjusted to suit the patient and the doctor. The nurse will be present throughout the examination to help the doctor and to make you feel more relaxed. If your clinic is in a large teaching hospital, there may also be a medical student or a postgraduate doctor (a registrar) present. If this worries you, have a word with the nurse or the doctor in charge.

You will be asked to remove your lower clothes and to

sit on the end of the couch. You then recline back and place your legs in the supports on either side of the end of the couch. This position is fairly comfortable as the supports are easily adjusted to suit women of different sizes if necessary. The position is initially embarrassing but the doctor and nurse will try to reassure you that all is well, and the embarrassment soon passes.

The important thing is to try and relax – the actual examination only takes a few minutes. The couch is raised a little and the doctor will insert a speculum so that he or she can look at the cervix. The doctor may then take another cervical smear. Having ensured that you are generally comfortable, the colposcope is then moved into position between your legs, just a short distance from the entrance to the speculum.

If there is any sign of vaginal discharge a swab can be taken. A small blob of cotton wool on the end of a thin wooden stick (like a cotton bud) is dipped into the discharge and then placed in a special culture medium and sent off to the laboratory for examination.

Washing the cervix

The cervix first is 'washed' with normal saline (a weak salt-water solution). All the solutions are applied using blobs of cotton wool on the ends of thin wooden sticks, similar to cotton buds. The saline solution helps to wash any mucus away, but more importantly, allows the gynaecologist to examine the blood vessels just beneath the surface of the cervix, since the wet cervical surface reflects light well. The blood vessels are shown in more detail in different coloured lights – especially in green light. Many colposcopes are fitted with coloured filters for this purpose which are operated by the flick of a switch.

When a woman is pregnant the cervix often appears 'blue' – this can be seen by the naked eye just as well as with the colposcope. It is not bright powder blue but a dusky reddish blue – due to the increased blood supply to the cervix and uterus necessitated by pregnancy. If you are pregnant when you go to the clinic, the gynaecologist will

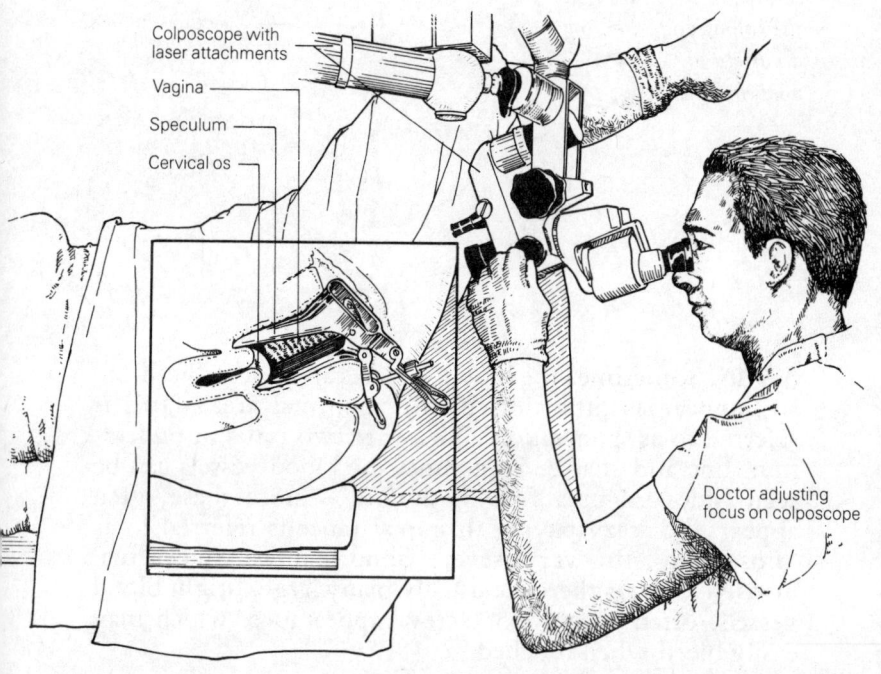

A colposcopy examination, using a colposcope with laser attachment. The Cusco's speculum in the vagina allows a clear view of the cervix (inset).

just apply the solutions but may not take biopsies. Once the gynaecologist is satisfied that a pregnant woman does not have invasive cancer, treatment can be delayed, but colposcopy may be arranged at intervals throughout the pregnancy, just to keep an eye on things. After the birth of the baby, the cervix will be less congested and treatment of the abnormal areas can be planned out.

The appearance of blood vessels

Mild to moderate abnormalities of the cervix producing mild or moderate dysplastic cells do not usually display any abnormal blood vessels. However, severe abnormali-

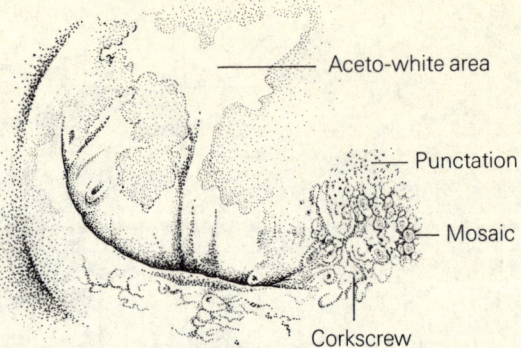

Blood vessels on the cervix, as seen through the colposcope, showing a variety of abnormalities.

ties do. Sometimes the blood vessels can be seen 'head on' and appear as little dots in the abnormal area – this is referred to as 'punctation'. There are two types of punctation, fine and coarse. Sometimes the blood vessels can be seen 'side on' in a fine meshwork – since these often appear like crazy paving this appearance is referred to as 'mosaicism'. In very severe abnormalities and actual invasive cancers there are usually many large, bright blood vessels, often with a 'corkscrew' appearance, which may easily bleed when touched.

Weak acetic acid solution

After the blood vessels have been examined, the cervix is then 'washed' again with a very weak solution of acetic acid, the sort of acid which appears in household vinegar. Applying it does not hurt. It tends to show up areas of abnormal cells as white patches called 'aceto-white'. As a general rule, to which there are often exceptions, the denser the aceto-white the more severe the abnormality, and the fainter the aceto-white the milder the abnormality. Why the cells should go white is the subject of some debate – a popular explanation is that the acetic acid dehydrates and blanches them. The acetic acid certainly make the fronds of the endometrial cells inside the cervical os (known as 'villi') stand out clearly.

The acetic acid solution is also very efficient at dissolving away blobs of cervical mucus which may still be obscuring the cervical os – the place which the doctor will want to see as clearly as possible.

The blanching aceto-white effect occurs after about one minute of 'washing' and passes off after a few minutes.

The upper limit

From the time the colposcopy examination starts and during the washing with saline and acetic acide solutions the gynaecologist will be looking for the edges of the transformation zone – this is very important indeed. He or she will be looking for the edge of the columnar endometrial cells, helped by the acetic acid which shows up the villi of the columnar epithelium. The edge of the transformation zone inside the external os will hopefully also be clearly visible. This means that any areas of abnormality can be seen completely, treated completely and easily followed up by examination with the colposcope. If however the upper limit of the abnormality cannot be seen clearly you will be advised to have a cone biopsy (see Chapter 5).

If the upper limit of the abnormality can be seen and the

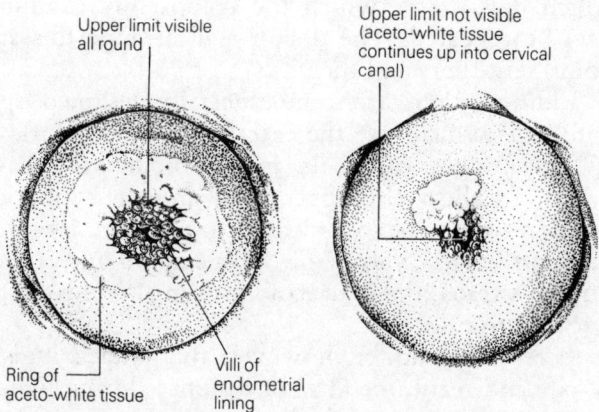

The upper limit of the transformation zone is searched for during colposcopy. Here it is seen in its entirety (left) and only partially (right). In the latter case, a cone biopsy would be necessary.

area of abnormality looks like pre-invasive disease, that is not an invasive cancer, then it can be treated by simple means – what is known as local ablative therapy (LAT), such as laser, cryocautery, hot cautery or cold coagulation, all of which are described in Chapter 4. Many of these simple treatments can be carried out in the colposcopy clinic and do not require admission to hospital.

Aids to viewing the upper limit

As you can appreciate it is highly desirable for the doctor to be able to see the upper limit of the abnormality and the edge of the transformation zone in the cervical os. In older women, especially after the menopause, the decrease in the levels of the female hormone oestrogen causes the transformation zone to shrink up the cervical canal, as the cervical os itself shrinks and begins to involute. In some younger women, oestrogen hormone tablets can be given to encourage the upper edge of the transformation zone to come down the canal, and for the cervical os to open up a little, to improve the chances of seeing the upper limit of any abnormal areas on the cervix. If this is suggested, you would be asked to take the oestrogen tablets for ten to fourteen days, after which the colposcopy examination would be repeated. The doctor will arrange this second appointment there and then.

In addition, there are some especially designed 'spreading' forceps which ease the external os open a little. This may be enough, especially in a woman who has had children, to allow the upper limit and the whole transformation zone to be seen clearly. In addition, by carefully adjusting the two 'valves' of the speculum and stretching the upper vagina, the gynaecologist can also encourage the cervical os to open.

If there is any doubt, however, the gynaecologist will play safe and recommend a cone biopsy during which the abnormal tissue beyond the limits of vision is removed.

Iodine solution

At this point in the examination, a weak solution of iodine

is then dabbed on and wiped over the whole surface of the cervix and upper vagina. This will show the outer limits of the abnormal area or areas. Normal cells contain sufficient sugar substances to react with the iodine and stain black. Abnormal cells stain honey brown and the limits can be easily seen. The iodine is put on last because a normal ectropian (see Chapter 1) will also stain honey brown, but will have been distinguished from abnormal cells by the examination with saline and acetic acid solutions.

Occasionally areas of abnormality encroach on to the vaginal epithelium (which is also covered in squamous cells). This will also be shown up by the iodine staining. These areas will, of course, also need treatment as well as the abnormal cervical areas.

Areas of cells which have previously been infected by the genital wart virus (HPV), in other words koilocytosis, give a characteristic ragged appearance when stained with iodine. Previous treatment using the freezing probe (cryocautery) can also cause small round areas which take up the iodine stain less well, so the doctor doing the colposcopy examination must know about any previous treatment to the cervix.

Biopsies

A biopsy is a small sample of tissue which is removed for examination in a laboratory. If, as is usually the case, the doctor can see the upper limit of the abnormal areas during your colposcopic examination, then a biopsy (or more than one) can be taken to help plan treatment. If the upper limit cannot be seen you are likely to be recommended for a 'cone biopsy', which is a more extensive procedure used actually to remove whole areas of abnormal cells (see Chapter 5), so there would be little point in taking an ordinary biopsy at the colposcopy clinic.

Biopsies are useful because occasionally the appearances of the blood vessels, aceto-white areas and the iodine staining may not give a true picture of the underlying abnormality and your doctor may want to double-check the diagnosis. In some cases the abnormal area may be worse than thought from its appearance through the colposcope, and in others it may well not be as bad. Most experienced colposcopists are right most of the time, but are always prepared for surprises.

If the cervical smear results correlate well with the appearances of the abnormal area only one or possibly two minute fragments of tissue (biopsies) need to be taken, but if there is a discrepancy, or large areas of abnormality need to be checked, then up to three or four biopsies may be required.

The minute fragments of tissue (biopsies) are nipped off from the surface of the cervix using very long thin biopsy forceps, which usually have a tiny beak-like end or little teeth for removing the tissue. Because they have to be passed alongside the colposcope, along the vagina to the cervix, they are very long – up to 60cm (2ft) and may appear frightening at first glance. However, removing the biopsies is usually painless, or if not, only causes a minor nipping-like ache for a second or two. The doctor doing the colposcopy will explain exactly what is happening and nothing will be done suddenly or without warning.

The little tissue fragments (biopsies) are placed in single pots, containing formalin solution to preserve them on the way to the histopathology laboratory. Each biopsy is labelled with its location, perhaps by comparing the cervix to a clock face, so that biopsies may be taken from, say, the 11 o'clock and 4 o'clock positions. If more than a spot or two of blood appears at the biopsy sites the area can be treated with a silver nitrate stick which soon stops any bleeding. Excess stain is mopped out with cotton wool, and you may be given a sanitary towel to wear after the colposcopy examination to prevent any stain from running down the vagina on to your underclothes – you may like to bring your own for this purpose.

Checking for warts

If you are known to have had warts of the vulva or have them at the time of the examination, then the vagina, vulva and anus will be inspected carefully. Through the colposcope even the tiniest wart (often not visible with the naked eye) can be detected and its position mapped out ready for treatment planning.

Checking the vulva

The vulva is also inspected with the naked eye and through the colposcope for abnormal areas. These may appear without staining as a purple-red patch or in some cases as a white area, known as leukoplakia. Again, abnormal areas will be shown up after applying the weak acetic acid solution. This is done very carefully indeed, as the solution can sting on the vulva.

Any abnormal areas may be biopsied, but this time a small injection of local anaesthetic is given before the biopsy is taken from the vulva. Abnormalities of the vulva are relatively rare but are on the increase (see Chapter 8) so the doctor or nurse taking cervical smears, and the doctor performing the colposcopy examination, will carefully inspect the vulva and look for suspicious areas at colposcopy.

After the colposcopy examination

Most colposcopy examinations, including taking the cervical biopsies, only take a few minutes to perform. Afterwards the couch is lowered, your feet are placed on the step and then you rise into the sitting position. You should do this slowly and then sit there for a minute or two while your balance returns and until you feel quite well, before bending down to get dressed.

As can be imagined most women are in a bit of a state of tension when they arrive for a colposcopy appointment and sometimes the sensations of the examination and biopsies can mix together to make them feel light-headed on rising. As the majority of colposcopy examinations are quite painless it is the mixture of worry and released tension which can occasionally cause fainting especially in people who have a tendency to faint in other situations, for instance, at the dentist. If you do feel a little dizzy on getting up you should lie back on the couch for a minute or two until you feel fully recovered. Nevertheless the vast majority of women jump up from a colposcopy examination without any problems at all.

Further appointments
Treatment may be offered at the first colposcopy visit but in some clinics a second appointment is given at the end of the examination so that the results can be explained and further treatment arranged. In other clinics the doctor will write to you with the results of smears and biopsy reports when they come through, and explain in the letter what treatment is recommended. You then telephone to make a further appointment for the treatment. If the recommendation is for cone biopsy, arrangements will be made for you to be admitted into hospital for this in the not too distant future.

Biopsy results

The fragments of cervical tissue taken at the colposcopy examination are 'pickled' in formalin solution and sent to the histopathology laboratory. These biopsies are then specially stained and set in blocks of paraffin wax. Extremely thin slices of the tissue are cut off using a very fine bladed knife (microtome) and placed on a microscope slide. These are examined by a specialist in histopathology (the study of the effects of disease on tissues), often in conjunction with the doctor who performed the colposcopy examination. The histopathologist prepares a written report which is filed in the woman's colposcopy/hospital records after it has been seen by the gynaecologist in the colposcopy clinic.

This process may take only a day or two but if the pressure of work on the laboratory is very heavy or there are staff shortages, then reports may take a fortnight or so to come back. An even bigger pressure of work usually faces the cytology laboratory and smear reports may be up to a month in arriving back at the colposcopy clinic.

The following explanations will help you understand what the histopathologist might find.

Koilocytosis

Occasionally the histopathologist reports only the presence of koilocytes (cells with wart virus infection changes). This may well have been suspected from the colposcopic appearances of the iodine staining. Many colposcopy clinics will offer treatment (local ablative treatment – LAT), to eliminate the areas of koilocytosis in view of the link between some types of wart virus and the development of pre-invasive cancers of the cervix. Often areas of koilocytosis will be coincidental with areas of other abnormalities – especially CIN (see below). Biopsies from actual warts on the cervix are reported as 'condyloma'.

The CIN grading system

The histopathologist will report the findings of your colposcopic biopsies according to the CIN grading system. CIN is an acronym for cervical intraepithelial neoplasia, which is a complicated medical way of referring to pre-

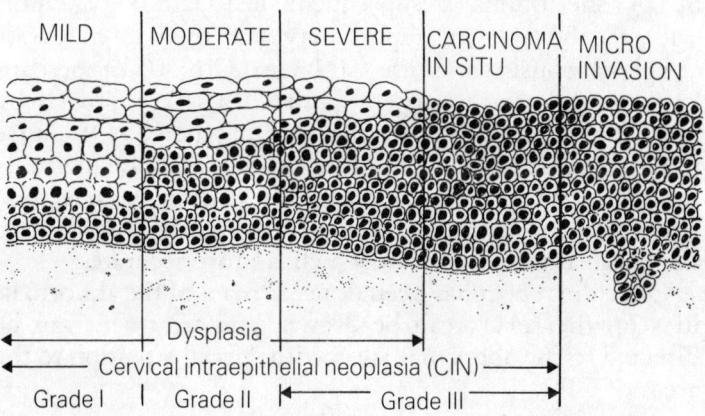

The changes on the cervical surface, as reported by the cytologist (dysplasia) from the smear, and the pathologist (CIN) from the biopsies.

cancerous abnormal cells in the surface layers of the cervix. Even doctors find it a bit of a mouthful and tend to abbreviate it simply to its initials.

The CIN grading system is not just based on the appearance of the cells, which is what the cytologist goes by when giving a class of abnormality on a smear report, but takes into account the depth to which the abnormal (dysplastic) cells have penetrated into the cervical epithelium. The degrees of depth, or thickness, are graded as CIN I, CIN II and CIN III.

CIN I, the least serious, is where the abnormal cells have taken over one third of the thickness of the epithelium; CIN II is where they occupy two thirds of the epithelial thickness and CIN III – requiring urgent treatment, but still completely curable – is where there is a full depth of abnormal cells but these have not yet penetrated the basement membrane. Full thickness CIN III used to be known as 'carcinoma in situ'. All these abnormalities carry a substantial chance if not treated, of developing into an invasive cancer, the risk being greatest with CIN III.

Occasionally a cytologist reporting on a cervical smear will try to correlate the degree of dysplasia seen with what he or she thinks a subsequent histopathology report will say. So a smear report may say 'mild to moderate dysplasia consistent with CIN I or CIN II' or perhaps 'severe dysplasia consistent with CIN III', followed by 'urgent referral to colposcopy recommended'. Of course the cytology report may not be entirely accurate in guessing the histopathology findings, but usually there is good correlation. Treatment, however, is usually based upon the histopathology report, which is more accurate.

Once the report has been done, a 'map' of the abnormalities on the cervix can be drawn, and treatment can be directed to the abnormal areas with special attention to the areas of CIN.

Depth of treatment

Under a microscope it can be seen that the surface of the

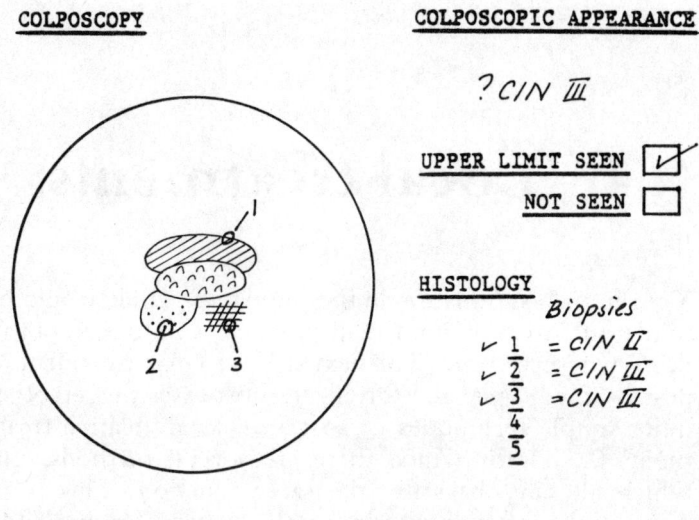

A 'map' of the abnormalities found on the cervix during the colposcopy examination, recorded by the doctor using a standard code. This map is sent to the pathologist with the biopsies for analysis.

cervix is not in fact completely smooth. There are little crypts which give the surface contours. The abnormal cells may occupy these crypts and therefore any treatment must destroy the tissue down to a level which includes the cells at the bottom of these crypts. This is very important when the problem is CIN III. Some colposcopy clinics will choose one type of treatment for CIN I and CIN II areas, and another, more powerful, type of treatment for CIN III problems. This is often treatment using the laser.

4 Local treatments

Your initial examination in the colposcopy clinic would be to identify areas of abnormality, if any, and to map out in detail where they are. The next step is to plan treatment to destroy them once and for all. In most cases this involves quite simple techniques of so-called 'local ablative treatment' (LAT) for which there are several methods, but which all have basically the same function. This is to destroy the offending cells in the cervix, leaving only healthy tissue in place. Almost all these treatments can be done in the clinic, or as day cases without having to spend a night in hospital, and, although they cannot said to be painless, they can be compared favourably to having a tooth filled under local anaesthetic at the dentist's.

There are no rules about what you may be offered in terms of local ablative treatment. The various techniques – laser treatment, cryocautery (freezing), diathermy, cold coagulation – are all described in detail in this chapter, and some clinics may have more than one of these techniques available, using whichever is most suitable to an individual case. Many colposcopy clinics use laser for all forms of CIN I, II and III; some use the cold coagulator for all types of CIN; some use laser for CIN III and cold coagulator or cryocautery for the rest. Still others simply use cryocautery for their main treatment.

Although the laser machine is very much more expensive than either the cold coagulator or cryocautery (both machines cost around £1,000), most units that want a laser now have one, either from NHS funds and/or local appeal. Currently several trials and studies are being conducted to compare one form of treatment with another to see which is the best, but many doctors in this field feel that the actual type of treatment used is not as important as the need for careful follow-up afterwards.

Menstrual periods

As is the case with cervical smears, it is best to avoid having local treatment on the cervix during the middle of your period, as the flow of blood through the cervical os may obscure the area to be treated. Again, light bleeding at the beginning or end of a period may be all right, but as previously, check with the clinic beforehand when you are given the date for your treatment. If you know roughly when your next period is going to be, make sure that it doesn't overlap your appointment, and if your period starts unexpectedly just before your appointment, telephone the clinic receptionist to change it, to avoid a wasted trip.

Laser treatment

The word 'laser' is an acronym for 'Light Amplification Stimulated Emission of Radiation', and it is basically a high energy beam of light. The carbon dioxide laser, most often used in colposcopy work, has its main beam in the infra-red – and therefore invisible – part of the spectrum. The apparatus which produces the beam for cervical treatment is about the size of a small desk, from which comes a metal arm attached to a colposcope. The generated laser beam is conducted along the arm so that it shoots out from the end of the colposcope into the area visible through it, vapourizing the abnormal cells at which it is directed. The power of the beam and the length of each laser emission can be varied, and the beam is fired using a foot pedal. Laser machines for this type of work cost between £30,000 and £40,000, and provide a highly effective treatment.

Laser treatment is often performed in the colposcopy

clinic and an appointment for it will be sent to you after your colposcopy examination. Laser machines may also be housed in general hospital day case departments, in which case you would be sent an appointment to attend as a day case (that is, having to attend only for a few hours), for laser treatment.

Preparation for treatment

During laser treatment you lie on the leg-supporting couch as for ordinary colposcopy. If the area to be treated by laser vapourization is small no anaesthetic is required as there is little pain. If the area is of moderate size then a local anaesthetic is injected into the cervix. If the area of abnormality is large, or if you are very nervous and found the initial colposcopy examination very unpleasant, the laser treatment can be performed under general anaesthesia, (fully asleep).

If general anaesthesia is chosen the anaesthetist will probably place a tiny needle in a vein on the back of the hand and tape it into place. The anaesthetic liquid is injected into the vein and you quickly fall asleep. When you are fully asleep a mask is placed on your face to maintain the anaesthesia for the five or ten minutes the laser treatment takes. The mask is connected to an anaesthetic machine which supplies the gases – often nitrous oxide (laughing gas) and oxygen.

A speculum is inserted into your vagina and your cervix is visualized. Iodine solution may be dabbed on the cervix to show up the extent of the abnormal areas on the cervix – the doctor wll have already checked the 'map' of the original colposcopy report and the areas of abnormality indicated by the histopathology reports.

Operating the laser

Once the anaesthetic, if any, has taken effect, the colposcope is lined up and the laser treatment begins. By pressing the control pedal, the doctor can shoot the laser either as a short burst or a continuous beam. The direction of the beam is along an ordinary visible light beam – often red or purple – which shows up on the cervix where the laser is targeted. When the beam hits the cervix it completely vapourizes a tiny area about 2mm square, and it is usually swept over the area to be destroyed until it has all been covered. The laser vapourization is then continued down to the desired depth in the cervix. If the abnormality to be treated is mild to moderate, say CIN I or II, the depth of treatment may not be as great as if there is a severe CIN III problem, which may be down to a depth of 8 to 12 millimetres.

As the cervical tissue is vapourized a certain amount of steam and smoke is created, sometimes accompanied by a smell of burning. To maintain clear vision of the cervix, and to prevent any unpleasant smell, a suction device is fitted to the speculum to evacuate the vapour in the vagina. To prevent any danger from reflected laser rays, the speculum is coated in non-reflective paint and the medical and nursing staff often wear protective glasses during the treatment.

After the laser treatment has been completed an antiseptic cream is often applied to the cervix to minimize the chance of infection.

Is laser treatment painful?

Some women undergo extensive laser treatment, chat away during it and then hop off the couch and go back to work the same day, having felt no more than a mild type of period pain. Other women find even the smallest laser treatment frightening and very painful. Some assessment and estimation of how you may react to laser treatment can be made by the doctor during the first colposcopy examination and the taking of biopsies.

If the area to be given laser treatment is large and deep, it is likely to be painful. Some doctors give each woman a pain-relieving tablet thirty minutes to one hour before treatment to minimize any discomfort. Some give a pain-relieving tablet after laser treatment and then suggest that you rest for a similar period. Some women will be selected for general anaesthesia straight away. If the injection of local anaesthetic is not sufficient, and you haven't eaten or drunk anything for some time previously, it is possible, although not always easy, to give you a general anaesthetic half way through the treatment. Some doctors have music playing in the background while they use the laser and their patients find this most enjoyable; one colleague of mine favours Mozart's Horn Concertos as highly suitable.

Laser treatment does present something of a doctor's dilemma. On the one hand, most women do not require general anaesthesia, which is one of its big advantages. On the other hand, no doctor wants a woman to find the laser experience unduly painful. A good discussion with each patient beforehand usually allows an experienced colposcopist to make the right decision.

Healing after laser treatment is invariably excellent, so that the cervix looks completely normal even when viewed closely a few months later. The success rate of this treatment is extremely high but careful follow-up is necessary so as to identify those few women who will have further problems.

Sexual intercourse after laser treatment
The gynaecologist in the colposcopy clinic will recommend a period of abstinence from sexual intercourse after laser treatment to the cervix (or indeed after any form of treatment to the cervix) while it is healing up. New cells will grow into the treated areas and be covered by new squamous cells which will be normal and not dysplastic. During this time of healing it is thought that sexual intercourse may traumatize and injure the cervix and that infection may possibly be introduced.

Some doctors also advise against using tampons during the healing period as they might also injure the delicate new cells.

Individual advice may vary but a period of abstinence of four to six weeks is quite commonly recommended. During the period of healing there may be considerable discharge passing down the vagina, often enough to cause some women to wear a sanitary towel – the light, press-on type is quite suitable. This discharge may occasionally be bloodstained. Before leaving the hospital after laser treatment you should make sure that you are quite clear that you understand what your doctor recommends about sex – this advice is often given in the form of a leaflet to take away and read at leisure.

When the scab which forms over the healing area breaks off spontaneously it may expose a small blood vessel which could cause prolonged, and on rare occasions, excessive bleeding. In such a case, you should contact the hospital and/or colposcopy clinic at once for advice and help, for which an emergency appointment is usually given.

Cryocautery

Cryocautery means destroying tissues using extreme cold – from the Greek words 'kryos', meaning cold, and 'kaustikos', meaning burning or corrosive. The cryocautery machine consists of a nozzle with a special cone which fits snugly into the external os and covers the outside of the cervix (ectocervix) for much of its surface. Gas such as nitrous oxide is released at high pressure and passed through the nozzle internally which has the effect of rapidly decreasing its temperature. The nozzle is attached to a handle which is connected in turn by a tube to the gas cylinder; the overall appearance is one of a large pistol. Each machine comes with a variety of nozzle shapes and sizes to enable different shapes and areas to be treated as well as possible. When the trigger is depressed there is a slight whooshing sound as the gas flows around the nozzle and lowers its temperature (down to about $-50°$ to $-70°$ C).

For cryocautery, a Cusco's speculum will probably be used to visualize the cervix. The end of the nozzle is carefully inserted into the cervical os and the rest of the nozzle gently applied to the surface of the cervix. The trigger is squeezed and the temperature of the nozzle rapidly falls. When a good ice-ball has been obtained around the nozzle the timing is started. The actual duration of freezing will be decided by the gynaecologist and will often consist of two freezing sessions with a period of thawing in between. To treat, CIN I or CIN II, a typical schedule would be three minutes' freeze, five minutes' thaw and three minutes' freeze again. (If the cryocautery is being used just to treat a benign ectropian which is causing too much watery vaginal discharge, then only one freezing session for a minute or two will be required.)

During the freezing you may well experience a dull central pelvic ache, similar to that of early period pains. This soon passes off when the treatment has finished although a couple of pain-relieving tablets, such as paracetamol, are often given afterwards to ensure a speedy return to comfort. Most women find the ache of the cryocautery easy to tolerate and no form of anaesthetic is required. Antiseptic cream is sometimes applied after treatment.

The same sort of period of healing follows after cryocautery as occurs after laser treatment. For the first two weeks or so there is usually a considerable volume of watery discharge along the vagina, which occasionally may be blood-stained. A period of abstinence from sexual intercourse will be recommended especially while you are experiencing the post-treatment vaginal discharge. Cryocautery sometimes leaves residual scarring on the cervix which is detectable with colposcopy and iodine staining subsequently. As with laser treatment, the success rate is very high, but follow-up is essential.

When will cryocautery be chosen?

Compared to a laser, a cryocautery machine is relatively cheap to buy and to maintain, and many gynaecology departments will have one. Cryocautery is often selected for the treatment of large cervical ectropia which are causing discharge and/or contact bleeding, such as post-coital bleeding, or for abnormal areas of the cervix with histopathological reports confirming only CIN I or CIN II is present. Occasionally it has been used to treat koilocytosis.

More serious CIN III areas are, however, usually treated with other methods, which can penetrate deeper than cryocautery to ensure that no residual abnormal cells are left behind, such as those in the bases of crypts. The usual treatment in these cases is vapourization. Cryocautery is only suitable when it is clear that the abnormal cells are confined to the area covered by the treatment nozzle. If the abnormal area covered the whole of the cervix and encroached on to the upper vagina, it would be difficult to ensure that all areas were covered with the cryocautery.

The cold coagulator

A cold coagulator machine consists of several probes with handles attached by a flex to a box the size of a large loaf of bread. At the end of each probe is a pad or nozzle. The small nozzles fit into the cervical os, whereas the round flat pads, approximately one centimetre across, are used for treating the outer cervix.

An electrical current is used to heat the end of the probes to a temperature which is usually 100° C, but may be higher or lower. It may seem odd to call something 'cold' which operates at the boiling point of water, but it is so-called because it is very much cooler than the 1000° C temperature used for old-fashioned hot wire cautery!

For this treatment, you will lie comfortably on the colposcopy couch, and a speculum will be inserted into your vagina to display the cervix. A little iodine solution can be dabbed on to the cervix to show the limits of the abnormal area. The pads on the end of the probes are applied for 20 seconds or so each in turn until the areas of abnormality have been completely covered and treated. Following this the cervix is covered with antiseptic cream.

The cold coagulator destroys the surface of the cervix by heat coagulation down to a depth which should remove all the abnormal areas in most cases, and this makes it very suitable for the treatment of koilocytosis, CIN I, CIN II and some areas of CIN III. While the pad is in contact with the cervix you will probably experience a central pelvic ache, similar to period pains. The pain quickly subsides when the pad is removed, but a residual ache may remain for a few hours which can be relieved with a simple analgesic such as paracetamol.

After treatment with the cold coagulator the cervix takes a month or two to heal up completely. When it has healed there will be no residual scarring and the area of treatment will be undetectable. During the first few weeks of healing there will be considerable mucus discharge down your vagina, which will occasionally be blood-stained. This discharge is often heavy enough for you to need to wear a sanitary towel. A sanitary towel is usually recommended rather than a tampon to reduce the chance of damage to the healing cervix. The gynaecologist will also recommend a period of abstinence from sexual intercourse for similar reasons, and to reduce the chance of infection. The success rate and the need for follow-up is the same as other forms of treatment.

Diathermy treatments and hot wire cautery

These treatments involve burning away the abnormal areas down to a selected depth using one of several systems. One uses a wire attached to a handle through which an electric current is passed. This heats up the wire to the desired temperature (ten times the boiling point of water), and allows the gynaecologist to burn away the abnormal areas.

A second system uses the ordinary diathermy kit used in everyday operations. This consists of an electrode wrapped around the thigh and a small metal probe attached to a handle. When a pedal is depressed a current flows through the two electrodes and burns the area in contact with the metal probe, down to the depth required. Another system uses a ball cautery with the other electrode consisting of a needle inserted into the cervix.

Performing the operation
All of these methods are performed under general anaes-

thesia (fully asleep). Since they are relatively minor procedures they are often performed as 'day cases' in hospital, which means that you would be admitted to hospital in the morning, having had nothing to eat or drink from the night before; you would have the operation, and then go home the same day. With day case surgery a heavy premedication injection before the operation is often avoided as this may make the woman too sleepy afterwards. The premedication can either be avoided altogether or reduced to a minor sedative with or without a substance to dry up the secretions in the mouth. You will be asked to sign a written consent form, as with any operation in hospital. This implies that you have had a thorough explanation of the procedure and understand what it involves. Make sure that you do get this explanation beforehand.

You will be taken from the ward (often a specially built day case ward) to the anaesthetic room. There a thorough check of identification is made to ensure the right patient is bought up at the right time. The anaesthetist will either give an injection of the anaesthetic solution directly into a vein with a syringe and needle, or tape in a little needle first into the vein on the back of your hand. The anaesthesia is usually maintained by a mask connected to a supply of nitrous oxide and oxygen. Sometimes a stronger agent such as halothane vapour is also added to the anaesthetic gas mixture during the operation.

After the operation some antiseptic cream is placed on the diathermied cervix and you are taken out to the recovery area to wake up fully. When you are completely awake you will be taken back to the ward or day case area and often be offered a very welcome drink (a cup of tea rather than a gin and tonic!) and allowed to get dressed when ready.

Some women bounce up straight away after a general anaesthetic and cannot wait to leave – others will feel rather sleepy for an hour or so. You should not drive a car after such an anaesthetic and it would be sensible for you to be picked up by your partner, friend or relative, rather than travel home alone on public transport. If you live far from the hospital or do not recover well from the general anaesthetic, or have concurrent medical problems which require observation, the doctor may suggest that you stay in hospital overnight and leave well recovered the following morning.

As with other forms of local treatments to the cervix it will take several weeks to heal and you may well be advised to avoid sexual intercourse while the healing is taking place to avoid trauma to the cervix and minimize the risk of infection. During the first week or two of healing there is often a heavy mucus discharge down the vagina which may occasionally be blood-stained. You should report any prolonged or heavy bleeding to the colposcopy clinic by telephone and seek their advice.

Follow-up appointments

Some gynaecologists will give a follow-up clinic appointment in a relatively short time after the local treatment, such as four to six weeks, to check that the cervix is healing well. However, the important check will be in the colposcopy clinic as much as four to six months after treatment. At this visit the doctor will take a cervical smear and make a thorough inspection of the cervix, not just the healing area, assisted by the application of the solutions described in the initial colposcopy examination. This check is to ensure that all the abnormal areas have been treated and that the cervix is healing well. It is quite likely that biopsies will not be taken as the cells from the areas of healing, called metaplasia, look too much like those of CIN I (see Chapter 3) to the histopathologist.

Further follow-up colposcopy appointments are often given as a matter of routine after local treatments, say after a further four or six months. At these visits a cervical smear will be taken and another examination performed with the colposcope. Any abnormal areas of the cervix which are seen at these visits will be biopsied, and any residual or new areas of koilocytosis or CIN will require further treatment. This is uncommon, however, as in the vast majority of women local treatment usually clears up the abnormality at first go.

Having said that, it cannot be emphasized too strongly how important the follow-up colposcopy checks are after any form of treatment. Although the treatments are highly effective a small percentage of women (around 5 per cent) will not be fully in the clear and all women need careful watching after treatment. When the colposcopy clinic is satisfied that all is well the doctor there will suggest that you just have cervical smears without colposcopy examinations in future follow-ups. Arrangements are usually made to have these at your general practitioner's surgery or family planning clinic. Some doctors will suggest moving to smears every year, while others will suggest that they are performed more frequently, such as every four to six months for the first year or so after treatment. Thereafter most doctors recommend annual smears for any woman who has had koilocytosis and/or CIN treated.

Insurance policies

Doctors in colposcopy clinics occasionally receive questions on how the diagnosis and treatment of cervical pre-cancers affect future life insurance policies. These are often related to acquiring a mortgage when moving flat or house.

It is sensible to make this sort of request in good time and in the formal written manner. It is usual for the insurance company to write to the colposcopy clinic doctor with a request for a brief medical report on the past treatment for CIN and it may ask for the doctor's opinion on the chance of the problem occuring again and/or the likely effects of the disease upon your life span. Before releasing any such information your doctor will require your written and signed consent that you give him full permission to release these medical facts to the named insurance company. Furnishing the report usually attracts a fee – the recommended fee for a short medical report at the time of writing is £13, although this, of course, can vary.

It must be emphasized that such a breach in patient–doctor confidentiality can only be authorized by you yourself in writing. Colposcopy doctors, like any other doctors, will not release any information about their patients without their permission.

It is impossible to predict the response of the colposcopy doctor on the chance of recurrence in any individual woman, and how this should affect life risks. However, a reassuring guide can be given from the reply by Dr Richard Reid at the Seventh Annual Meeting of the Australian Colposcopy Society held in Melbourne in 1984 to the question of a patient seeking a life policy after receiving treatment for CIN III. Dr Reid felt that women who have negative colposcopy examinations and negative cervical smears in the first year of follow-up could be placed within one of the lowest risk categories for subsequently developing cervical cancer. He quoted from a multi-centre survey conducted by Dr R. M. Richart and colleagues reported in the American Journal of Obstetrics and Gynaecology in 1980, which followed 3,000 successfully treated women for up to fifteen years and demonstrated a recurrence rate of less than one per cent.

5 Cone Biopsy

If you are recommended to have a cone biopsy rather than one of the local treatments described in the previous chapter, it will be for one of the following reasons. The first is because the upper limit of the abnormality cannot be seen by colposcopy (see Chapter 3); the second, that your doctor had a suspicion during the colposcopy examination that there had been micro-invasion or actual invasion of the basement membrane by the abnormal cells. The third, and most rare, reason may be that you haven't actually been examined in a colposcopy clinic as such because your gynaecologist has no access to one, so is obliged to treat all women with a severely abnormal smear in the same rather drastic way – either with cone biopsy or hysterectomy.

The aims of cone biopsy

The cone biopsy operation can both help find out what the problem is and remove the abnormality at the same time. In other words, it may be curative as well as diagnostic. As a result, the word 'biopsy' may be misleading in some circumstances.

A cone of tissue is cut out of the cervix to include the whole of the abnormal area and, in particular, to get above the abnormal area inside the cervical canal as it enters the endometrial cavity (see Chapter 1). The cone of tissue is sent to the histopathological laboratory for analysis to see if the abnormal cells have invaded through the basement membrane and to see if all the areas of abnormality have been completely excised.

Admission and preparation

Cone biopsy operations are not performed as day cases; they always involve a general anaesthetic and a few days' stay in hospital. However, in some places you may be admitted into hospital on the day of the operation, while in others you will have to come in on the day before. Some surgeons do not like performing cone biopsies during a period, because they think the risk of extra bleeding is increased at this time. If you are expecting a period to coincide with your admission into hospital for cone biopsy you should telephone the hospital for advice, in order to avoid a wasted journey.

In hospital you will be examined by a doctor to make sure you are fit for general anaesthesia and then you will be asked to sign a consent form, after you have ensured as far as possible that you are fully informed of what the procedure entails and have had a good chance to have any questions answered.

A plastic band containing a card with your name, age and hospital number is attached around your wrist. This is part of the stringent checking procedures on patient identity that are carried out in the wards, anaesthetic rooms, operating theatres and recovery areas. You will not be allowed to eat or drink for at least six hours before the operation to ensure that your stomach is empty during the operation and when you are waking up from the anaesthetic.

Premedication

About an hour or so before the expected time of the operation a premedication injection is often given. Individual anaesthetists have their own preferences for premedication mixtures, although the basic recipe usually consists of a pain-relieving and anxiety-reducing drug of the morphine type, combined with a substance to dry the secretions of the mouth and throat. A popular combination involves a type of opium that most people find very comforting and relaxing.

A cone biopsy will usually be performed as part of a schedule of gynaecological operations that lasts all morning or all afternoon, and will be an operation of about 20 minutes amongst others that can last from five minutes to three hours. Sometimes operations go faster or more slowly than originally planned, so it may be difficult for you to be given a precise time for yours. The nurses on the ward will be very busy getting women back from recovery and sending patients up to the theatres, but will probably be able to keep the waiting patients informed of how the operation list is going for time. However, after the premedication is given, the curtains will be pulled around your bed and you will be disturbed as little as possible, so that you can lie there thinking pleasant thoughts or have a little doze. On the other hand, some premedication injections do not contain heavy narcotics or sedatives, so if you find yourself awake and not sleepy when the theatre attendants come to take you to the theatre, you should not be alarmed.

The anaesthetic

The anaesthetic is usually started (or 'induced', as anaesthetists say) by an injection into a vein on the back of the hand or in the arm. This causes you to fall quietly asleep in less than a minute. Often a fine needle is inserted into a vein on the back of the hand, and attached to the needle are two plastic wings so that the needle can be held in place with a small piece of tape – this often referred to as a 'butterfly'. The butterfly allows the anaesthetist to give further injections into the vein during and after the anaesthetic without having to prick the vein several times.

The anaesthetist will also give a pain-relieving injection into the vein to ensure a comfortable and smooth recovery from the anaesthetic. Sleep will be maintained by a mask supplying nitrous oxide and oxygen gases, to which can be added more powerful anaesthetic gases during the operation if necessary. If the cone biopsy is being combined with laparoscopy, sterilization or other procedure in the abdomen the anaesthetist may well give a muscle relaxant and take over your breathing by placing a tube in the windpipe and connecting this to a mechanical ventilator, but this is not usually necessary for the cone biopsy by itself. Some anaesthetists will insert a drip into a vein on your arm when you are asleep. This leaves a very thin plastic tube in a vein, through which injections and fluids can be given.

The anaesthetist may well wish to monitor your heart beat throughout the operation. This can be done by feeling the pulse frequently; nowadays many anaesthetists use monitoring machines. Before you are asleep small sticky pads attached to wires are placed on your chest. In theatre these connected to an electrocardiographic machine (ECG) which measures the pulse and displays the heart beats on a small visual display unit (VDU) at all times. Similarly, your blood pressure can also be measured automatically by machines which give the anaesthetist a digital readout.

When the anaesthetist is satisfied with your condition, you are wheeled into the theatre on a trolley and, using the canvas stretcher, lifted gently on to the theatre table and the poles removed. Your legs are then lifted into supports on either side of the operating table. Your vulva is then cleansed and you are covered in sterile towels.

Removing the affected tissue

The gynaecologist will paint iodine solution on to the cervix to show up the outer limits of the abnormal areas as indicated on the colposcopy report. Using a thin scalpel blade, he or she will then cut out a cone of tissue around the external os to include all the abnormal areas. To prevent bleeding before cutting into the cervix, injections of lignocaine and adrenaline can be given into the cervix.

CONE BIOPSY

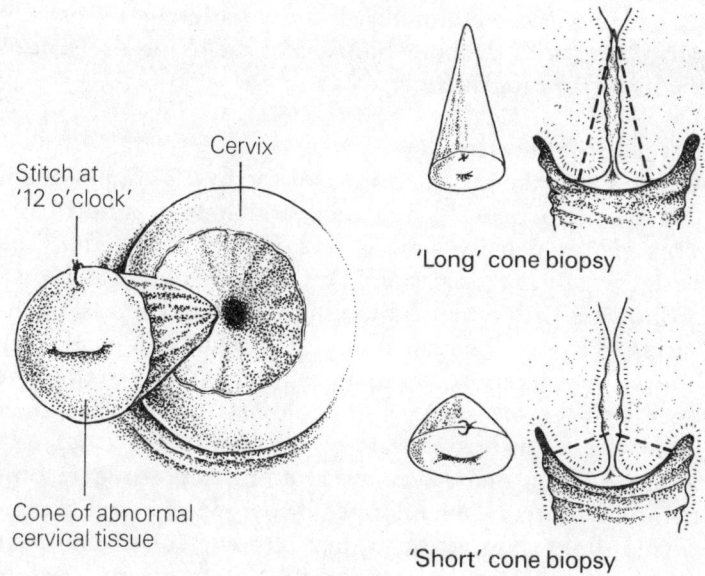

'Long' cone biopsy

'Short' cone biopsy

The cone biopsy aims to remove all the abnormal tissue and leave as much normal cervical tissue as possible.

When the cone has been removed a little stitch is placed in it at the '12 o'clock' position to orientate the histopathologist when he or she receives it in the laboratory. The raw areas of the cervix, which may have some residual bleeding, are then treated with hot cautery and antiseptic cream.

If injections have not been placed in the cervix, soluble stitches are inserted instead particularly in the '9' and '3 o'clock' lateral positions where the main blood vessels come in. Any stitches placed in the remaining cervix, however, will distort the shape of the cervix and can make it difficult to examine it completely with the colposcope afterwards. Some gynaecologists place a ribbon gauze (soaked in lubricating, antiseptic proflavine cream – which looks and feels like custard) into the vagina against the cervix to discourage bleeding. This gauze is usually removed the following day.

A scrape of the endometrial cavity (curettage) is usually performed with the cone biopsy and the tissue also sent to the histopathologist for analysis.

After the operation

When you wake up, and often for the first 24 hours or so, you will experience a dull ache similar to a period pain. This is not usually serious and will be relieved by an analgesic tablet or injection. The main problem for a small proportion of women is bleeding from the cut area of the cervix. This can happen at any time while it is healing up but is most likely to occur in the first 48 hours after the operation – so many gynaecologists insist that their patients stay in hospital after cone biopsy for at least 48 hours of post-operative observation, and some recommend 72 hours or even longer. Most women will experience a slight amount of vaginal bleeding for several days after the operation but it should not be heavy. Before leaving hospital you will be told what to do if you do experience heavy bleeding – this usually means telephoning the hospital and returning immediately. Sexual intercourse should be avoided until healing of the cervix has occurred and advice will be given on this.

Follow-up visits

Many women will leave hospital after two or three days and this will often be before the histopathologist's report on the cone biopsy tissue and the endometrial scrapings (curettings) will have been received. Some gynaecologists will see a woman a week or two after the cone biopsy in the out-patient clinic to convey the contents of the report, others will delay this for up to six weeks and then, at the same time, examine the cervix to check that healing is going well; if all is well sexual intercourse is often resumed after the six week appointment.

Some gynaecologists write to patients when the report

is received saying that all is well and arrange to see them in the colposcopy clinic for follow-up in about four months' time. After cone biopsy all women will be followed up in the colposcopy clinic for cervical smears and colposcopy examinations. The timing of the visits may vary from clinic to clinic, but a typical schedule would be, the first follow-up colposcopy examination four months after the operation, and the second visit six months after the first, etc. When the gynaecologist is satisfied in the colposcopy clinic you can then be followed up by cervical smears only at specified intervals – these can be performed by your general practitioner or family planning clinic in most cases.

Other post-operative problems

By and large there are no problems following cone biopsy other than the bleeding mentioned above. If stitches of catgut are inserted these will dissolve after about ten days and small bits of them might be seen floating in the bath. Occasionally their dissolving is accompanied by slight bleeding. Menstrual periods usually return on time but occasionally may be heavier or lighter for a month or so.

On rare occasions infection in the womb and pelvis may follow cone biopsy or old inflammation may be stirred up by the operation. The symptoms would be pelvic pain, spells of fever and a vaginal discharge which is usually foul smelling. This is treated by rest in hospital and/or at home and courses of antibiotics.

In very rare circumstances the cervical os (see Chapter 1), becomes blocked after this operation and the menstrual fluid is unable to escape during the period. At period times, there is pain but no bleeding. If this happens, you should inform your doctor who will arrange for you to return to hospital for examination, which will reveal a blocked os. This can be easily opened up again. However, if periods stop after a cone biopsy, you should also consider the possibility that you might be pregnant.

Cone biopsy, fertility and pregnancy

In theory the cone biopsy should remove the external os

and unless there is good healing with a return to the normal mucus needed for sperm capacitation (see Chapter 1), fertility would be affected. In practice this is not usually the case and the vast majority of women who were fertile before cone biopsy will be fertile afterwards. The modern cone biopsy operation, which is colposcopically directed, will aim to remove the absolute minimum amount of the affected cervix and therefore minimize the chance of functional damage to the cervix. However, if you are trying for a baby after cone biopsy and experience difficulty in conception, help should be sought, sooner rather than later, initially from your general practitioner.

If extensive, cone biopsy can damage the internal os (see Chapter I), and this may cause the cervix to open up when the baby enlarges after the twelfth to fourteenth week of pregnancy (cervical incompetence). The modern colposcopically directed cone biopsy operation will keep tissue damage to a minimum and will protect the internal os as much as possible, thereby reducing the chances of this. However, any woman who has had a cone biopsy should book for antenatal care as soon as she knows she is pregnant. The obstetrician in the antenatal clinic will find out details of the cone biopsy and examine the cervix to see if there are early signs of the os opening up. He can decide whether it is necessary to have a cervical stitch insertion under general anaesthetic, after twelve or thirteen weeks of pregnancy.

This stitch is often called after Professor Shirodkar, an Indian doctor who in 1955 introduced an operation that was then made simpler, by McDonald in 1963. Telling women they need a McDonald's in this day and age can often lead to thoughts of a hamburger rather than a cervical operation. Either way, the stitch is removed painlessly without the need for anaesthetic at about 38 weeks of pregnancy and the mother usually goes into labour naturally soon afterwards.

Opinions vary a good deal on the problem of cervical incompetence. It is not very easy to decide whether in individual cases a woman needs a cervical stitch or not after cone biopsy. On the one hand, no one wants to give any woman a stitch if she does not need one as there is a very small risk of miscarriage, but, on the other hand, if a stitch is omitted and the cervix is very weak the woman will miscarry towards the middle of pregnancy anyway, often without very much warning, and the baby will be lost. With a cervical stitch in place, the baby is safely 'locked in' to the uterus, so many obstetricians will recommend cervical stitches for all women after cone biopsy, to be on the safe side. Others will examine the cervix every week or so and then select you for a stitch if the os shows any signs of opening. In any case, with colposcopically directed cone biopsies now being performed, the amount of tissue removed is much less, reducing the risk of cervical incompetence accordingly.

Hysterectomy

Occasionally, women who need a cone biopsy also have other gynaecological problems, such as very heavy periods (menorrhagia). Indeed, you may have gone to your family doctor or gynaecologist with one of these problems and a routine smear taken at this initial examination may have been found to be abnormal quite coincidentally. After colposcopy examination, the possibility of performing a total hysterectomy (removal of the womb and cervix) could be discussed with older women who have completed their families and are also having treatment for a problem such as menorrhagia.

There is a considerable difference in the two operations in terms of stay in hospital, recovery times, anaesthetic and operative risks, as well as emotional factors, and so the decision to perform a hysterectomy rather than just a cone biopsy will not be taken lightly. In this situation, a woman would have a colposcopy examination first to exclude any possibility of invasive cancer and to see if the abnormal areas on the cervix encroach on to the upper end of the vagina so that the whole abnormality should be removed at hysterectomy.

Cone biopsy reports

The vast majority of reports show that the area of abnormality did not include any sign of invasion through the basement membrane (see Chapter 1) and was completely cut out, so that no abnormality was left behind. However, even if your biopsy report is clear, you will still need the same follow-up as anyone else – that is to say, further colposcopy in the first year after the operation, and annual smear tests thereafter until 65 years of age. However, a few women will have a different report. The area of abnormality may not have been completely removed and an area could remain on the outside of the cervix (ectocervix), or on the inside of the cervix (endocervix). The report may show that there has been invasion of the abnormal cells through the basement membrane for a few millimetres. This is called 'microinvasion' and is discussed in the next chapter. Finally, and most rarely, there has been deep invasion of the abnormal cells through the basement membrane. This is called invasive cervical carcinoma

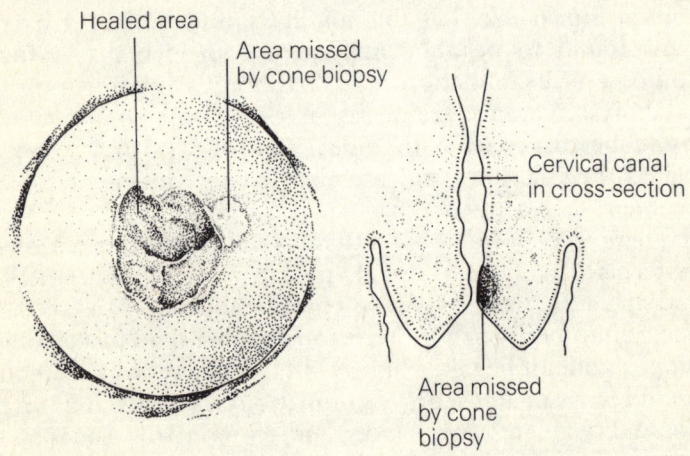

The abnormal tissue may be inadequately exised by a cone biopsy, leaving an area on the ectocervix (left) or endocervix (right).

(cancer) and is also discussed in the next chapter.

Further treatment if abnormal cells remain

If the area of abnormality was not completely removed on the outside edge (ectocervix) the area will be visible with the colposcope and may be suitable for local ablative treatment such as with the laser, or a form of cautery (see Chapter 4). If the area of abnormality was not completely removed high inside the cervical canal (endocervix) this will not be visible and another, deeper cone biopsy will be required.

Nevertheless, it is reassuring to know that the great majority of cone biopsies performed after colposcopy examinations have mapped out the area of abnormality will remove the whole abnormality at one go. Only a very few women will require further treatment.

Cone biopsy using laser

There is now considerable interest in using a laser cone biopsy as an outpatient procedure instead of laser vapourization (see Chapter 4). The laser cone seems to be straightforward and effective and has the advantage of providing a cut-out cone of tissue for analysis. In some women the cervix may display a mixture of abnormalities (see Chapter 3) with CIN III in and around the canal and a CIN I and/or CIN II abnormality around the outside (ectocervix).

Instead of cutting away a large cone of cervical tissue using a scalpel to include the whole area of CIN I and CIN II, a smaller cone can be cut out using the laser beam (see Chapter 4) to include the CIN III area, and then the CIN I and CIN II areas could be removed down to the desired depth using conventional laser treatment. This keeps the actual damage to the cervix down to an absolute minimum.

6 Cervical cancer

Although this is a book about the prevention of invasive cancer by screening and early treatment, it would not be right to ignore the fact that many women do unfortunately have to face the fact of microinvasive or invasive cancers of the cervix. But they still stand a high chance of being cured if the disease is caught early. Tumours of the cervix can be removed from the pelvis by surgical operations or destroyed by radio therapy. Radiation treatment can be extremely effective, using external beams of high energy rays, along with the insertion of radio-active rods into the uterus, which will destroy the adjacent tumour.

Obviously prevention is better than cure, and everybody hopes that if more women come forward for regular cervical smears, we will be able to prevent these cancers from developing. The vast majority of women who currently develop invasive cervical cancer have never had a cervical smear. But even if you do have regular smears, it is important that you come forward for a check-up as soon as the symptoms of a suspected tumour appear. These may be bleeding after intercourse, a blood-stained, watery discharge, bleeding in between periods, or bleeding vaginally after the menopause (when periods have stopped altogether). The earlier the treatment is started, the better chance there is of surviving.

If the cancer has just started to invade the cervix (microinvasion), it is possible to minimize treatment, but once the cancer has deeply invaded, treatment must be extensive (radical).

Microinvasion

Following cone biopsy described in the previous chapter, in a very small proportion of women, the report from the histopathological laboratory may state that the abnormal cells have penetrated through the basement membrane (see Chapter 1) for a very short distance only – a matter of two or three millimetres or so. This is the first sign that the abnormal cells on the surface of the cervix are becoming malignant and starting to invade the cervix.

There is considerable debate about what is microinvasion and what is true invasion – in other words, a malignant tumour. The treatment of microinvasion is essentially simple, while the treatment for invasive tumours is much more extensive. Before discussing treatment options, the gynaecologist will have had a discussion with the histopathologist and looked at the slides of the stained tissue. The gynaecologist will be concerned to note the actual depth of invasion, whether it has occurred in more than one place and whether the tumour cells have entered the tiny blood vessels and lymph channels.

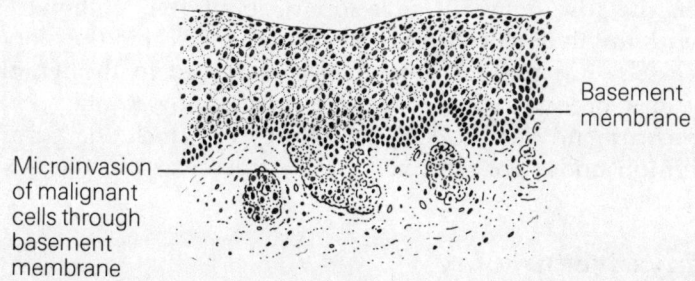

In microinvasion, the cancer cells have just penetrated the basement membrane by a few millimetres.

Treatment

The treatment options available would be cone biopsy alone, or with subsequent hysterectomy, or radical hysterectomy. On the one hand the gynaecologist will want to keep treatment to the minimum amount of surgery, on the other he or she will not want to risk under-treating a malignant tumour.

In discussing treatment with a woman who has micro-invasive disease the gynaecologist will take many factors into consideration – the state of the tumour and the situation of the woman herself. There is obviously a variety of situations which can occur. For example, she may well be young, say 25 years of age, with no children as yet, and would like a family eventually; the depth of invasion may be only one or two millimetres with no invasion of the blood vessels or lymph channels. In her case the gynaecologist may well feel that the cone biopsy is treatment enough at the moment, and she will be followed carefully with the colposcope. At the other end of the spectrum the woman may be 45 years of age, having already had children, and completed her family. She may have heavy periods which are very painful. Her depth of invasion may be three or four millimetres. In that case a form of hysterectomy (removal of the womb and cervix) would be highly satisfactory to clear up the period problems and the abnormal cells at the same time. Another situation might be that the depth of invasion is about five millimetres with involvement of the lymphatic channels and the blood vessels – in this case the chance of spread to the lymph nodes becomes likely and the gynaecologist may well recommend a radical hysterectomy in which the pelvic lymph nodes are removed – this is described in the next section.

Invasive tumours

When the biopsy has confirmed that the abnormal cells have invaded into the deeper tissue of the cervix the gynaecologist must find out exactly how far the tumour has spread. The pattern of spread follows one or more of several paths.

Sometimes the tumour will be discovered when it is still confined to the cervix. It may appear on inspection as a bleeding ulcer – giving symptoms of a blood-stained vaginal discharge, bleeding between periods, bleeding after sexual intercourse, or bleeding after the menopause. With all these symptoms the cervix needs to be inspected and a cervical smear and/or colposcopy examination performed.

If further invasion occurs the tumour may invade down the vagina, up into the uterus and out to the ligaments on the side of the cervix and uterus which hold the uterus in place (these ligaments and their muscle fibres are called collectively 'the parametrium'). In very advanced cases the tumour may invade through to the bladder in front of it, causing the urine to become blood-stained; or it may invade through to the structure behind it – the rectum – causing the passing of blood with faeces.

Staging

The extent to which invasion has occurred when it is discovered is mapped out in a system called staging, numerically I to IV; with I being early invasion and IV being very extensive invasion. Stage II is divided into (a) and (b) subgroups; in the IIa group the invasion extends from the cervix to the upper part of the vagina and in IIb the tumour has started to invade the parametrium (the ligaments and muscle fibres on the side of the uterus and cervix) but the tumour has not reached the side wall of the pelvis (stage III). When the tumour has invaded the rectum (lower large bowel) and/or the bladder it is described as stage IV disease. Stage IV disease also includes situations where the tumour has spread to the spine or chest or anywhere outside the pelvis.

Lymph nodes and lymphatic channels

The various organs of the pelvis – uterus, bladder, rectum, vagina – have a network of lymphatic channels, as do other parts of the body such as the breast, the neck and the arms. Along these channels flows an oily liquid called lymph. To say that the lymph channels act like sewer pipes

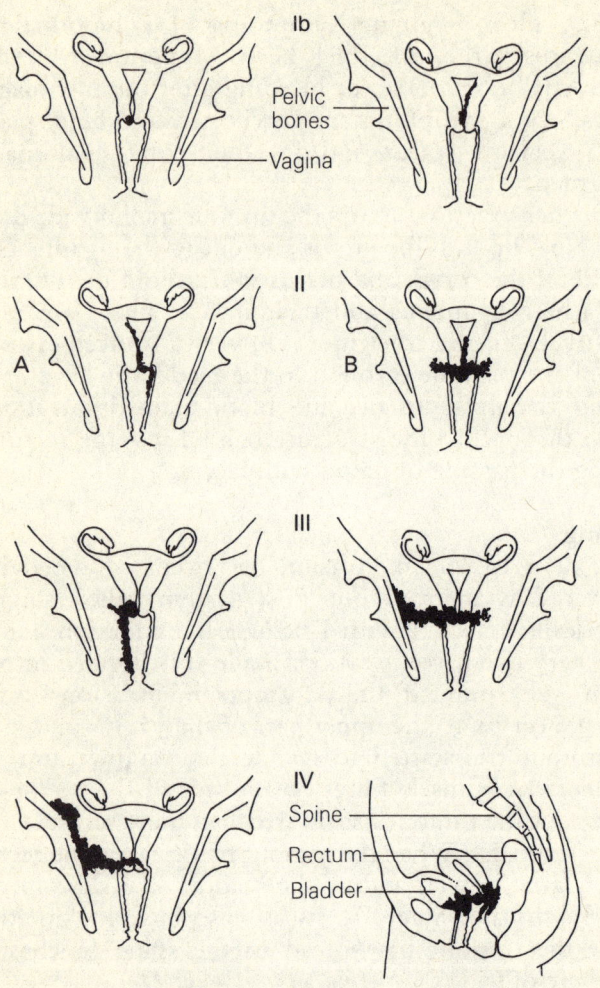

The stages of invasive cervical cancer:
Ib *The cancer is confined to the womb*
IIa *It has encroached on to the top of the vagina*
IIb *It has invaded the tissue around the cervix (parametrium)*
III *There is extensive involvement of the vagina and/or invasion out to the bones of the pelvic side wall*
IV *The cancer has invaded beyond the pelvis and/or adjacent organs, such as the bladder and rectum.*

in an house or street is a bit strong but in many ways the analogy is true – the lymphatic system conducts away unpleasant material – especially bacteria and other organisms of infection. Within the network are junctions called lymph nodes, which produce special cells called lymphocytes. Many of these are adapted to perform special tasks – in particular they form much of the body's immune defence system against infection. When the immune system is injured or suppressed the body loses its ability to fend off even simple infections. Some of the lymphocytes actually ingest (eat) bacteria and other types of infective organisms, preventing them spreading and multiplying.

The lymph nodes and lymphatic system play a very important part in the body's ability to prevent cancers forming and to restrict the growth and spread of cancers once they have become established. When a tumour has started to spread the tumour cells may well travel along the lymphatic channels and settle in the lymph nodes.

The lymphatic channels and lymph nodes draining the cervix and uterus are situated mainly around the large blood vessels along the back and sides of the pelvis. Any woman who has an invasive tumour of the cervix is at risk of having tumour cells in the lymph nodes of the pelvis, and any treatment planned for her must either remove or destroy these tumour cells. Some types of invasive tumours do not spread to the lymph nodes until the very late stages, but other, more wild, types of tumour spread to the lymph nodes at a very early stage of invasion.

The lymph nodes of the pelvis are connected to a chain of lymph nodes further up in the abdomen and these are connected to those in the chest. Very wide spread of the disease into the abdomen and chest is possible either along the interconnected lymphatic channels or by tumour cells being carried by the bloodstream along the veins and arteries. As a broad generalization it could be said that tumours of the cervix tend to remain in the pelvis and do not spread around the body as frequently or as early as do tumours of other organs – however, there are exceptions and the gynaecologist will want to check as far

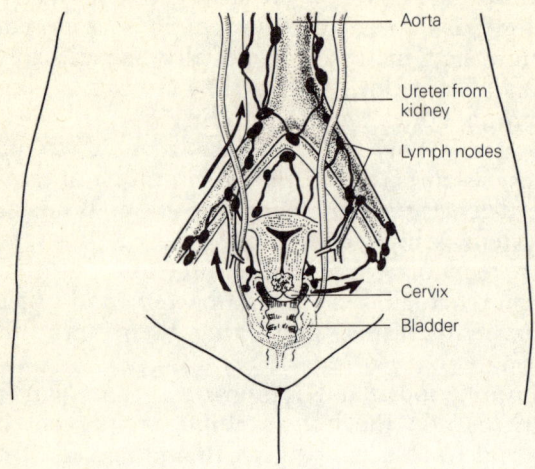

The lymphatic channels which drain tumours of the cervix pass out to lymph nodes on the walls of the pelvis around the arteries and veins.

as possible for distant spread before planning treatment.

Pre-treatment tests

In addition to the usual checks of the blood for anaemia and levels of chemicals and enzymes the gynaecologist will request certain special tests. An electrocardiograph (ECG) is usually performed routinely to check the heart before any surgery is contemplated. A chest X-ray will be taken to see if there has been any spread to the lungs or bones of the chest. An intravenous urogram will be arranged – this is known as an 'IVU', but it may also be referred to by its old name of 'IVP' (intravenous pyelogram), and in the USA, as 'KUB' (kidneys, ureter, bladder).

IVU

Before the IVU a woman is given an injection of a dye which is opaque to X-rays (radio-opaque) into one of the veins of the arm. After a few minutes the kidneys filter out this dye which collects and concentrates in them and then passes down the ureters to show up the bladder outline. If the tumour has invaded the bladder, or compressed it, or squashed one or both of the ureters this will be shown on the IVU.

Other tests
In some units the size and extent of the tumour may also be measured using various types of imaging machines, in particular the Computerized Axial Tomography (CAT) scan and the Nuclear Magnetic Resonance (NMR) scan. The CAT scan is produced by reforming a large number of small X-ray images arranged in a circle around the woman into a TV-type image by a computer (computer-enhanced image). The NMR scan is produced by placing the woman in a strong magnetic field and, using a computer, forming a TV-type image of the various tissues in her body from the different ways each tissue reacts in the magnetic field. Tumours appear differently from the surrounding normal tissue.

In both cases 'slices' of pictures through the pelvis can be obtained. Ultrasound scanning, the type that is extremely useful in maternity work, is not used very much in cervical cancer treatment.

Examination under anaesthetic (EUA)
If there is any doubt about the extent of tumour the gynaecologist may wish to examine the woman while under general anaesthesia. This offeres an opportunity to check the vagina and the parametrium on both sides, to feel for extension of the tumour in the parametrium and look for extension of the tumour down the vagina.

In addition the bladder will be checked by inserting a lighted telescope and looking at the lining (cystoscopy), and the rectum will be checked by inserting another type of lighted telescope (proctoscopy).

Planning treatment

Once the stage of the tumour has been worked out then

treatment can be planned. As far as possible the choice of treatment will be tailored to the needs and situation of the woman. There are three types of treatment for invasive cervical cancer: surgery, radiotherapy and chemotherapy with cytotoxic drugs. Some women may need combined treatment, for example surgery followed by radiotherapy, or chemotherapy followed by surgery.

Surgery: radical hysterectomy

This operation to remove the tumour along with the rest of the womb is often referred to in Europe as 'Wertheim's hysterectomy', after the Viennese surgeon who first performed it in the early 1890s, and a 'Meig's hysterectomy' in the USA, after a famous surgeon at Massachusetts General Hospital in Boston. Radical hysterectomy may be used to treat stage I and early stage II tumours.

It is performed under general anaesthesia. During the operation drugs to relax the muscles are given to the patient to help the surgeon, so the anaesthetist will place a tube in the windpipe connected to a mechanical ventilator to take over the woman's breathing movements (see Chapter 5). The operation takes two to four hours.

During the operation the uterus, cervix and tumour are removed. To ensure that the tumour is completely taken away a margin of normal tissue is cut away around it. This involves removing the tissue on either side of the cervix (the parametrium) and the upper part of the vagina.

One of the main problems for the surgeon is that the ureters, the small tubes bringing urine from the kidneys on either side in the loins down to the bladder which rests on the front of the cervix and uterus, pass through the parametrium, quite close to the cervix and tumour before entering the bladder in front. The ureters are therefore separated out with time-consuming care. The lymph nodes along the lymphatic channels draining from the cervix and its tumour are also removed. The groups of lymph nodes are attached to the major blood vessels of the pelvis, so considerable care is taken to remove them all and not to damage the adjacent blood vessels and nerves.

If the woman is still having periods, the ovaries can be left in place, or moved to the upper abdomen out of range of any subsequent radiotherapy. If the woman is post-menopausal (after the change of life) the ovaries can be removed to ensure that they do not subsequently undergo cancerous changes themselves.

Because the bladder can be bruised during this operation a catheter is often left to drain the urine for a few days after the operation, but this is by no means always so.

Recovery

The first day or so after this operation is usually uncomfortable, and strong pain-relieving injections are often given and gratefully received. The bowel often stops working for a day or two but usually resumes normal function soon after and by the third or fourth day the woman will feel much better. When the bowel stops working it tends to dilate and causes the belly to swell. If this happens fluids are usually given by the intravenous drip, as drinking stresses the bowel even further. Passing flatus (wind) is usually a good sign that the bowl is starting to work again, although it is often embarrassing for the patient to admit the good news!

Following radical hysterectomy, women usually go home after one or two weeks – depending on variables such as whether the woman lives alone, how old she is, or concurrent medical problems. Resuming normal duties at home usually takes a further fortnight and those women with jobs should not try to return before six to eight weeks, perhaps going part-time for the first week or two, to ease back into the swing of it.

The surgeon will often wish to see the woman in the clinic six or so weeks after the operation and check that all is well before recommending a return to work, sport, sexual relations, aerobics, etc.

The histopathological report

Before the woman leaves hospital the report from the histopathology laboratory will have been received. This will inform the gynaecologist how big the tumour was, how aggressive it appeared under the microscope in terms of cell differentiation, whether the lymph nodes were involved with tumour and whether the tumour was completely cut out, so that the edge of the tumour was surrounded in normal tissue. If the tumour is not surrounded by normal tissue, the histopathologist will report 'positive margins'. If these are discovered, and/or the lymph nodes are involved, and/or there is a very aggressive appearance under the microscope (poor differentiation of the cells), then the gynaecologist may recommend extra therapy such as external beam radiotherapy and/or chemotherapy. However, it is reassuring to know that in the vast majority of cases the single operation will cure the cancer.

Before leaving hospital the woman will have the findings of the histopathology report discussed with her and for the majority of women this will mean the 'all clear'. However, even if the 'all clear' is given, very careful follow-up will be carried out over the next ten years.

Radiotherapy

There are two main types of radiation treatment given and women who are selected for radiotherapy may have a mixture of the two. The first type is 'external beam' treatment (teletherapy) and the second type is internal treatment inside the uterus and vagina with isotopes (brachytherapy). In both cases the high-energy radiation is carefully directed at the tumour and destroys cells that are growing. Radiotherapy may be used in all stages of cervical cancer.

External radiotherapy
This consists of high-energy ray treatment to the pelvis and parts of the abdomen. Radiotherapy can be produced by a variety of high-energy machines. The treatment is not given all at once but in so-called 'fractions' over a period of weeks. For example, the dose of radiotherapy could be given in four daily treatments each week for six weeks.

Side effects

By dividing up the total dose the side effects are kept to a minimum. Organs which are very sensitive to radiotherapy such as the kidneys will be shielded after a certain dose of radiotherapy has been reached. Initially some nausea is often experienced but this can be controlled with tablets if necessary. Later on the bowel may be disturbed and any diarrhoea caused can be counteracted again with tablets. Over the area of treatment the skin may become reddened – just like suntanning before the skin goes brown.

The bladder may also be disturbed causing a form of cystitis but this usually settles down by itself. In a few women, the lining of the large bowel and bladder may be thinned by the radiotherapy and they may occasionally experience some fresh bleeding even after the radiotherapy treatment has finished. This will be checked out by the doctors and will usually settle down without special treatment. However, any bleeding in the urine and/or with bowel motions should be reported immediately.

The radiotherapy treatment received is measured in units called Grays. However, one hundredth of a Gray is called a centiGray, and this term is often used in preference to a Gray because a centiGray is the same as one 'rad', the term for the unit used previously. A typical total dose would be between 4,500 and 5,500 centiGrays (cGys or rads).

Internal radiotherapy

This consists of placing radioactive isotopes inside the uterus and around the cervix so that the tumour can be given a lethal blast of radiotherapy from very close quarters. Isotopes give off mixtures of radioactive particles α(alpha), β(beta) and high-energy γ(gamma) rays. Many isotopes disintegrate quickly and are of no use in medicine. For many years radium was used widely because it decayed over a very long time and gave off a steady emission of radiation. Nowadays Caesium 137 is used. It, too, decays at a slowish rate (not as slow as radium) but it is preferred because it is a safer source and is less hazardous to the medical physicists, and other medical and nursing staff.

Techniques vary somewhat but the basic idea is the same. The woman is given a general anaesthetic, or an epidural anaesthetic, in which she remains awake but with the pelvis anaesthetized by an injection of local anaesthetic in the back, around the nerves leaving the spinal column. The cervix is opened up with dilators (small rods of increasing thickness) and a thin hollow tube is placed in the uterus which can take the radioactive isotopes. Against the cervix (and, of course, the tumour) are placed either cubes or ovals in which, again, can be placed the Caesium isotope. These are held in place with packing gauze. The isotopes are then inserted, and, using a Geiger counter to measure radiation, the bladder and the rectum are checked for excess radiation. If too much radiation is given to the bladder or rectum a hole may be burnt into these structures, so if there is too much leaking into them, the isotope sources and/or the packing material are skilfully moved to correct this. Great care and skill are employed in getting the positioning just right to avoid these problems. Often X-rays are taken to check that the position is correct.

After the anaesthetic has worn off the woman is taken to a special ward with lead screens to protect the nurses from radiation. The isotopes are left in place for a calculated length of time – often around 24 hours – and then the sources and tubes are removed. The procedure is usually repeated for two or three treatments, often one week apart.

This system gives a large dose of radiotherapy to the tumour in the cervix, often in the region of 10,000 cGys, and this big dose will kill off all but very large or very radio-resistant tumours.

The woman may feel some nausea with treatments and some discomfort in the pelvis when the tubes are in place; this is relieved by either tablets or injections. There may also be similar bowel and/or bladder disturbances. After treatment the vagina may be dry and usually the use of a lubricant is recommended to ensure that intercourse is comfortable.

Chemotherapy

Some young women have very aggressive tumours, which look 'wild' (undifferentiated) under the microscope, and are at very high risk of rapid spread to the lymph nodes and beyond. For these women some gynaecologists are trying treatment with cytotoxic drugs given by injection into the bloodstream to augment the radical hysterectomy operation – this has recently acquired the name of 'neo-adjuvant chemotherapy' because the drugs are given at the beginning of treatment as an adjunct to surgery. Cytotoxic drug treatment, however, for very advanced or recurrent cancer of the cervix has not yet been consistently successful but new drugs and new ways of giving them are being tried.

Follow-up

After radical hysterectomy or radiotherapy the woman will be seen in the clinic quite frequently in the first year. After a year or two clinic follow-up visits will be spaced out – moving towards annual visits. At follow-up visits any strange symptoms can be reported and looked into. The woman is examined for any signs of recurrence, particularly in the vagina and on the vulva; some gynaecologists will take a smear from the vagina and check it with the colposcope if necessary.

The outlook

The chance of survival and living a normal life (the 'outlook' which doctors refer to as the prognosis) after treatment for all women with a variety of stages of invasive cervical cancer is about 50 per cent. Although this is a rather depressing fate for those who suffer from the cancer, it may be a little consolation to know that it is a much better chance than with some other forms of cancer, such as lung cancer.

For women with early stage cancer of the cervix (stage I), the outlook is very good, with 80-90 per cent surviving at least five years after either radical hysterectomy or radiotherapy. Recurrent disease after five years is not common and the great majority of these women will survive beyond ten years, after which time many gynaecologists would say that they are cured and discharge them from follow-up clinic visits.

The majority of women with stage I disease will be aged between 55 and 65 years; however, there is a small but increasing group of women between 25 and 45 years of age who are developing invasive disease. Some of these are suffering from tumours which are particularly aggressive. The histopathological appearance of their tumours under the microscope is especially wild and the performance of the tumour can be one of rapidly fatal spread. In particular very early spread to the pelvic lymph nodes is found, followed soon after by involvement of the rest of the abdomen and chest. Conventional treatment may be unable to stop the disease in these women and the body appears to have little or no immunity, or at least very poor resistance to its rapid dissemination. In this situation the 'neo-adjuvant' type of chemotherapy would be used.

Women with stage II, III and IV invasive cervical cancer will, in the vast majority of cases, be treated with radiotherapy. In the best units women with stage II cancer of the cervix can expect a 60 per cent five-year survival rate. In the advanced disease, the prognosis is unfortunately poorer – a 25-30 per cent chance of five-year survival in stage III disease and no more than 10 per cent in stage IV.

As with many cancers the earlier the diagnosis the better the prognosis and outlook. Hopefully an increasing number of women will be treated in the pre-invasive (CIN) phase of the disease and thus prevent it from becoming invasive cervical cancer, and needing any radical treatment. This, of course, depends upon an effective screening policy.

7 The causes of cervical abnormalities

The exact cause of cervical cancer has not yet been discovered with certainty, but we now know a great deal about associated factors, and the pieces of the jigsaw seem to be fitting together. There have been a lot of medical surveys which have highlighted the groups of women at special risk, but to be effective, a screening programme has to include both high- and low-risk groups.

The way cervical cancer develops, with its pre-invasive stage, offers a tremendous opportunity to treat it before it becomes invasive and a risk to life. As we learn more about what causes the abnormalities in the first place, better advice can be given about prevention.

Sexual intercourse

It has been known for over a hundred years that women who have never had sexual intercourse do not develop cervical cancer. This suggests that a carcinogen (something which induces cancer) or a co-carcinogen (something that contributes to the development of cancer) is transmitted to a woman by the man during intercourse. This has led to a hunt for the 'male factor' – a search which has been going on for some time, and which has led down many blind alleys, but which now seems to be on the right track.

One early theory that seemed promising arose in the 1960s, when several reports from gynaecologists working with Jewish women in the USA noted that they had a relatively low incidence of cervical cancer, and suggested that this was due to their husbands' ritual circumcisions. It was thought that there may be a carcinogen in smegma, the secretion under the foreskin of the penis, which would not be present in circumcised men, and therefore, by definition, not present in Jewish men. However, subsequent studies of other groups looked at the effects of circumcision but couldn't confirm its protective effect, and no carcinogen was found in smegma. It is likely that the Jewish women originally studied in America fell into a low-risk group for reasons which had nothing whatever to do with circumcision (see later).

Even so, this did not rule out that men could be a factor in cervical cancer, and the hunt continued. Workers in Australia and the United Kingdom angled their attack on the possibility of a carcinogenic protein carried in semen – the mixture of fluid ejaculated during a man's orgasm, consisting of spermatozoa, secretions from the prostate gland, testes and seminal vesicles. (They also thought that the cause might be mutant spermatazoa.) However, this suspect protein could not be a natural protein carried by all men – it had to be a so-called 'rogue' protein, acquired by infection. This would explain why not all women who have had sexual intercourse develop cancer of the cervix – in fact, only a relatively tiny proportion do. And the most likely candidate for a transmittable 'rogue' protein is a virus.

Virus infections

A simple view of a virus is that it consists of a stripped down cell nucleus which can enter the nucleus of a normal cell, take over its control and force the cell to do its will. In some cases this will mean causing the cell to go into virus production, in others it will cause the cell to secrete normal or abnormal products in large measures; curiously, in others it will cause the cell to self-destruct, and in the case of a few viruses cause the cell to become cancerous. There are thousands of viruses already identified but only a handful are as yet known to produce cancers directly. Bacteria, parasites, fungi or yeasts are not usually associated with the direct cause of cancers and so it is unlikely that simple vaginal infections such as thrush (candida), Gardnerella, trichomonas, etc. (see Chapter 3) are likely to be part of the cancer process.

So far there is no evidence that AIDS (acquired immune deficiency syndrome), caused by HIV (human immuno deficiency virus), which can be transmitted during sexual intercourse, is a direct cause of cervical cancer. Of course, study of HIV has only been carried out for a relatively short time in the United Kingdom since the recognition of the AIDS disease here in 1982. More time is needed before any sure statement can be made about the HIV and cervical cancer, but one connection may be found in the spread of cervical cancer through the lymphatic system and other routes.

It is now established that a proportion of people who have been infected with HIV will have impairment of their immune system (especially that provided by the lymphatic system) and these people may therefore have less resistance than normal to the spread of cancers as well as of infections. It is just possible that those women, especially young women, who have rapidly spreading cancers of the cervix may have some form of suppression of the normal immunity and that this suppression is related to a viral infection such as those of the HIV type. It is now known that women whose immune systems are suppressed, either naturally or with drugs, are at high risk of developing CIN. In some studies the incidence of CIN amongst women whose immune systems are artificially suppressed by drugs following kidney transplants is as high as 10–20 per cent. It is quite impossible to make any firm statement concerning HIV and AIDS in general at the moment – most workers currently in this field suggest that any statements they make now are only true to the end of the week.

There are, however, two sexually transmitted viruses which have come under considerable suspicion and scrutiny – genital herpes and the genital wart virus. Although there is little strong evidence to date that herpes is a definite carcinogen or co-carcinogen, the finger is currently being pointed at the genital wart virus – human papilloma virus (HPV).

Human papilloma virus (genital wart virus)

It was suggested in 1977 that wart virus infection of the cervix might be a precursor of CIN. Recent studies have shown a strong association between genital infections with the HPV wart virus and the development of pre-invasive and invasive cervical cancers. A large proportion of women with CIN abnormalities have concomitant HPV infection of their cervixes, and a large proportion of young women with vulval warts also have warts on their cervix. A substantial number of these have areas of CIN.

In a North London study in 1983 of women with vulval warts, over one third also had CIN on their cervixes; in addition, one third of the partners of a group of men with persistent warts on the penis also had evidence of CIN.

Another study showed that 65 per cent of the male partners of women with CIN III had penile warts that were not recognized until examined under a microscope. Another 1983 study found that more than half of 620 cervical biopsy specimens from women with CIN or invasive cancer also showed evidence of HPV infection, and suggested that 'flat' type warts were more frequently associated with severe pre-cancers than the usually papillary wart.

Guilt by association is not true confirmation of cause, but the presence of genital warts and/or evidence of HPV infection of cervical cells must place a woman in a very high risk group for CIN.

The human papilloma virus is a small 'DNA tumor virus' and six or so of its 42 different types are associated with infection of the genitalia. HPV type 6 and HPV type 11 have been found in conjunction with pre-malignant abnormalities, whereas type 16 is associated with CIN and invasive cancer. In invasive cancer HPV type 16 becomes part of the host chromosome.

In one study, 85 per cent of women with CIN I which progressed to CIN III had evidence of HPV type 16 infection.

HPV has been found in laboratory specimens of cervical cancer, preserved from as long as 30 years ago, by hybridization techniques.

To try to demonstrate that HPV is part of the cause of cervical cancer rather than just being associated with it the kidney capsules of specially bred mice with no natural immunity have been infiltrated with tissue from the cervix which was then experimentally infected with HPV. It was found that malignancies resulted.

HPV and other genital cancers

There is an increasing incidence of women with CIN developing similar abnormalities of the skin of the vagina (VAIN – vaginal intraepithelial neoplasia), the vulva (VIN – vulval intraepithelial neoplasia) and the skin around the anus. Gynaecologists are now talking about a 'field change', that is to say that the skin covering the cervix, the vagina, the vulva, down to and including the anus, is all at risk from the same malignant processes. There is now evidence of similar premalignant abnormalities seen in the rectum (the lower large bowel connected to the anus) of homosexual men (known as RIN – rectal intraepithelial neoplasia, which is classed in similar stages to CIN – RIN I, II and III). One study showed that 75 per cent of RIN III sampled contained HPV type 16. Similar studies have shown that the same is true of VIN and VAIN (see Chapter 8).

The suggested role of HPV in cervical cancer

It is now suggested that human papilloma virus is harboured in the cervical transformation zone (see Chapter 1) after transmission during sexual intercourse in women and girls at risk. The area where the HPV is housed in the transformation zone may particularly help the entry of

HPV into the cells and then initiate the process of change to abnormal pre-cancerous cells (intraepithelial neoplasia – CIN), along with other co-carcinogens such as the breakdown products from cigarette smoke. This fits in with other factors such as the age of commencing sexual intercourse, multiple sexual partners and so on.

HPV and men

Of course this immediately brings the question to mind, what about men? It has been recognized in the last five years that while a woman may not seem to be at risk perhaps because she has not had many sexual partners, if her partner has many sexual partners he brings the risk to her. Unfortunately many men have no idea whether they are carrying HPV; if they are infected they may well have 'sub-clinical warts' – that is to say they are not visible with the naked eye and can only be seen with a colposcope and acetic acid staining. Men with visible warts should go promptly to a sexually transmitted diseases clinic (or Department of Genito-Urinary Medicine as they are now called) for treatment.

Early sexual intercourse

Many surveys have suggested that the majority of girls' and young women's first experiences of sexual intercourse are without using any form of contraception – it is only later that some protection from pregnancy is used. Some doctors think that venereally transmitted organisms are likely to be passed on during this time. The HPV could be transmitted in this way and be harboured in the transformation zone containing susceptible cells (see above). Whether this is a correct assumption or not, evidence from many studies performed in a variety of countries does suggest that adolescent sexual intercourse increases the risk of developing cervical cancer.

Smoking

It has been known for some time that cigarette smoking

increases a woman's risk of developing cervical cancer, although exactly how it happens is not known. What is known, however, is that nicotine and other products from tobacco are selectively secreted in the cervical mucus and it is quite possible that these act as co-carcinogens in the initiation or promotion of cervical cancer.

A recent survey amongst women in Atlanta in the USA showed that smokers had a risk of CIN III more than $3\frac{1}{2}$ times greater than that of non-smoking controls. The risk appeared to be dose-related in that with heavy smokers the risk of CIN III was as high as 12.3 times that of non-smokers. The findings held good even when age, number of sexual partners, age at first intercourse and oral contraceptive use were taken into consideration.

Many epidemiological surveys in the past suggested that women who developed cervical cancer belonged predominantly, but by no means exclusively, to the lower socio-economic classes, in which the proportion of women who smoke is much higher than in the professional classes, the exception being amongst the health care professionals, in which nearly 50 per cent of nurses smoke (about three times the proportion of women seen in similar professional employment). It is possible that the effects of socio-economic class on this disease are made worse through smoking rates as well as the age at early sexual intercourse.

Childbearing

It has also been established for some time that having children is associated with an increased risk of developing cervical cancer, and is also associated with a decreased risk of developing cancers of the breast, ovary and endometrium (lining of the uterus). It is not clear how the risk is increased, but a woman who has had children has obviously had sexual intercourse and that will give her a higher chance of developing cervical cancer than a woman who has never had sexual intercourse (and will never develop cervical cancer). Some doctors have also suggested that during pregnancy the cervix may be placed at greater risk of developing cervical cancer. At this time most women develop a cervical ectropian (see Chapter 1) in which the endocervical cells are more exposed on the cervix, a state which may persist after delivery of the baby. This could make the cervix more vulnerable to a venereally transmitted infection such as HPV. This physiological ectropian persists after pregnancy and occasionally long after weaning takes place.

The oral contraceptive pill

A similar situation occurs in many women who are taking the oral contraceptive pill. A proportion of these will develop a small ectropian (cervical erosion) and may, in theory, be more vulnerable to genital wart (HPV) infection. What is not known is whether this type of ectropian in an adult is as liable to contract HPV infection as it is in an adolescent or teenage girl. It is also not yet known whether the cells of an ectropian induced by pregnancy or oral contraceptive are as vulnerable as the cells undergoing change in an adolescent.

Although one study has suggested that long term oral contraceptive use increased the risk of abnormal cells when compared to the intrauterine contraceptive device (IUD or coil) there is not enough evidence to say which type of contraceptive may reduce the risk of abnormal cells forming. The study contained a number of variables and cannot be considered as conclusive. We await many more studies to examine this question more extensively – especially now that the amount of oestrogen in oral contraceptive pills has been greatly reduced over the last decade, which may reduce the amount of cervical ectropian produced.

The number of sexual partners

It has been known for a long time that promiscuity has an influence on the risk of cervical cancer in that women with a large number of sexual partners are more at risk than relatively monogamous women. This is understandable if a venereally transmitted infection such as HPV is really part of the cause. What has recently emerged is that the female partners of very promiscuous men are also at greater risk – again indicating that infection may be a cause.

'Safe sex' practices, such as the use of condoms during intercourse and reducing the number of casual sexual partners, may well lessen the risk of developing cervical cancer.

Is mild dysplasia an acute viral infection?

It has been well recognized that a significant but probably decreasing proportion of cervixes containing biopsy-confirmed dysplasia will return to normal after a certain length of time. Surveys have shown a return to normal in from as low as 28 per cent to 54 per cent of women (depending on the criteria for selection of the sample studied). Without sophisticated DNA and nuclear analysis, it is very difficult to differentiate between acute HPV infection and low grade CIN. In one 1981 series from a researcher called Meisels (who was credited in 1977 with the early recognition of HPV as a potential co-carcinogen) it is suggested that up to 70 per cent of low grade CIN abnormal areas were, in fact, only the effects of acute HPV infection. This, of course, may partly explain why some low grade CIN abnormalities return to normal. Old wart virus infected cells (koilocytosis) present a problem for the doctor – to treat or not to treat? Will it regress spontaneously? Is the infection from the dangerous type 16 human papilloma virus? In favour of always treating koilocytosis is the knowledge that it may be of the type to cause CIN and that follow-up in the group of women who predominantly suffer from it may be difficult or impossible for long periods in every case. (This is because they tend to be mobile, urban young women between 20 and 35, who may move addresses frequently, and may not receive or may ignore, pleas for follow-up appointments.) A recent group of women with koilocytosis only (that is, showing no abnormal cells yet), followed up by colposcopy examinations at the Middlesex Hospital in London showed that only 20 per cent regressed to normal while 3 per cent proceeded to CIN I and a staggering 45 per cent to CIN III. Other workers suggest that koilocytosis is unlikely to regress at all. Many doctors in Britain and the United States recommend a 'search and destroy' mission against koilocytosis for fear that it may progress to CIN without detection. The development of a vaccine against HPV infections might also offer some protection in the future.

It is not easy to be certain which categories of abnormalities will regress to normal, stay static or progress to more serious abnormalities. It is impossible to say how long the interval between progression from CIN I to CIN II to CIN III will take in individual cases, and it is also quite impossible to identify when, or by what stimulus, CIN III changes from pre-invasive states to become an invasive cancer. A lot of research into this is being carried out, particularly in the United States, and much attention is being given to something in the pre-invasive abnormal cells which stimulates new blood vessels to help it invade the basement membrane.

It used to be commonly taught that the interval between the pre-invasive stage, that is, CIN, and the development of invasive cancer could be as much as 20 years. But recent reports have cast doubt on this and in some patients the progression can be a matter of a year or so, or even months. However, much of the data currently available has been produced by busy colposcopy units working in inner city areas such as central London, and is quite possible that their statistics concerning CIN and invasive cervical cancer may be different from those obtained in other parts of the country, especially the more rural areas. Nevertheless there is considerable agreement in findings between the major colposcopy units in the large conurbations of Britain and America, and remarkable similarities in the performance of the disease.

In one project from Scotland, for example, 131 women with CIN III were studied. Invasive cancer developed in 35 per cent of these women after twenty years and in only 5 per cent did the CIN III regress spontaneously. Of the ten women in whom the original diagnosis was made by small biopsy, nine (90 per cent) developed invasive cancers. The following assessment of progression/regression rates is contructed from the data currently published, much of it obtained from inner London colposcopy centres:

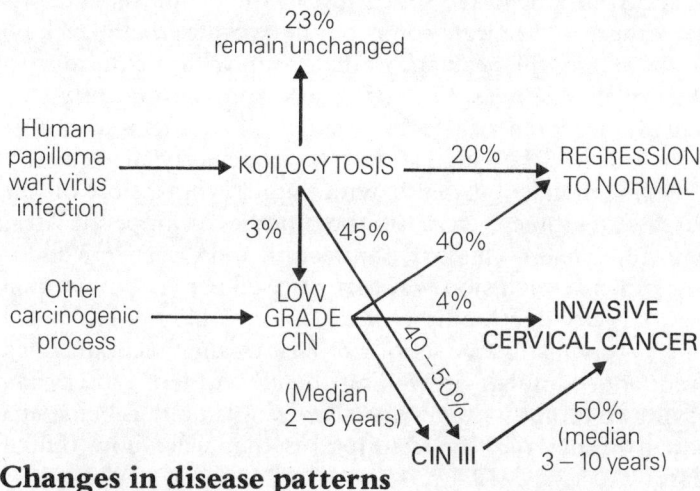

Changes in disease patterns

In 1983 centres on opposite sides of the Atlantic, one in Buckinghamshire and the others in Massachusetts and Tennessee, noticed changes in the occurrence of cervical abnormalities which cut across previously established risk associations.

The British centre noted from a retrospective analysis of the previous fifteen years an increased pick-up rate of abnormal smears greater than that for Britain as a whole. It had more than doubled in previously unscreened women (5.8 to 12.9 per 1,000 smears) and trebled in those who had been screened before (0.9 to 3.6 per 1,000 smears). The pick-up rate had increased in all age groups, but especially in women under 40. They had noted that there was a significant increase in population in their area of Buckinghamshire, especially in the younger age groups, with an upward shift of social class. This was contrary to the previous belief that lower socio-economic groups are most at risk from cervical cancer. One possibility was that the high mobility in the areas resulted in an influx of people who had had multiple sexual partners.

In the American report of 130 women with cervical cancer 25 per cent had a short interval of less than three years from a negative smear test to the diagnosis of cervical cancer. Although some of the women were over 60 years of age, the peak age in the group with rapid progression of disease was 30 to 35 years, and, significantly, the usually accepted risk factors, such as low socio-economic class or child bearing, were not particularly in evidence. Of the nineteen patients with rapid progression of the disease, eighteen were of the middle or upper classes, seventeen had no history of infection and three were childless. Their conclusion was that since 25 per cent of women with rapidly developing cervical cancer could not be singled out by any distinctive set of risk factors, they recommended frequent – annual – screening for *all* women, rather than trying to target women who were singled out as being at a much higher risk by assumptions that were now out of date.

8 Associated abnormalities

Other areas of the genital tract – vagina, vulva and skin around the anus – may also develop abnormalities related to those in the cervix. These possibly have a similar cause. In the early 1970s gynaecologists and pathologists in the United States of America noticed an increase in the number of women with pre-invasive cancerous changes on the labia (outer lips) and other parts of the vulva. The skin covering the vulva consists of squamous epithelium similar to that covering the cervix, the vagina and the skin around the anus. The pre-malignant changes on the vulva and in the vagina were examined under the microscope and classified in a similar way to cervical abnormalities, that is, VIN (vulval intraepithelial neoplasia) and VAIN (vaginal intraepithelial neoplasia) with the I, II and III divisions.

The age factor

Whereas preinvasive and invasive cancers of the vulva and vagina had previously been seen in relatively older women, over 50 years of age, there has been an increasing number of younger women found to have VIN and VAIN – especially in the 20 to 40 age groups. Similar findings were reported from other North American centres and more recently from the United Kingdom.

Relationship to CIN

A large proportion of the young women with VIN/VAIN were also found to have CIN and this has given rise to the idea of a 'field change' – that is to say that the skin surface from the cervix, down to the vagina, all over the vulva and the skin around the anus (all made up of squamous epithelium) is at risk from cancerous change, probably with the same causal agents. The risk factors of women with VIN/VAIN are similar to those with CIN.

As with CIN I, the changes of VIN I could be those produced by an acute viral infection by the genital wart virus (HPV), and some VIN I abnormalities have been shown to go away of their own accord. However, a substantial proportion progressed to VIN II and then VIN III and to invasive vulval cancer, if not treated.

Symptoms

About half the young women with VIN did not have symptoms, and nearly all women found to have VAIN did not have any symptoms at all. These women were picked up during screening for CIN, that is to say, their doctors noticed abnormal areas while taking a cervical smear. The other half of women with VIN mostly complained of itching and/or a purple or dark red area on their vulvas.

Investigation

When an abnormal area of the vulva and/or vagina is found it is examined with the help of the colposcope (see Chapter 3). It is examined thoroughly first and then a weak solution of acetic acid is applied very carefully (the vulva is much more sensitive than the cervix and without care the acetic acid solution can sting). As with CIN, abnormal areas of the vulva will show up with a distinctive appearance recognizable to the doctor. A biopsy is taken but this time a little local anaesthetic is injected into the area with a fine needle. If the area of abnormality is widespread multiple biopsies will be needed and these will be taken under general anaesthesia. Once the areas of abnormality have been mapped out and the degree of change in the cells assessed then treatment can be planned.

Treatment
If a large invasive cancer is found the treatment will be radical surgery in which the vulva is removed along with the lymphatic nodes of both groins. If there is just a small area of microinvasion the surgery can be much more limited. The gynaecologist will assess the degree of risk in each case and tailor treatment to suit the woman and her age and circumstances.

Choosing the treatment of the pre-invasive abnormalities known as VIN I, VIN II and VIN III is not so easy. Obviously the treatment needs to be kept to the absolute minimum while still destroying or removing the abnormal areas completely. As large areas of skin may undergo pre-malignant change when one small area is treated, an adjacent area may subsequently start to change.

Treatments have varied between using the carbon dioxide laser, electrocautery, chemotherapy with a paste containing the cytotoxic drug 5-fluoruracil, limited surgical removal and a skinning vulvectomy in which the top skin of the whole vulva is removed and replaced by a split skin graft from the skin of the thigh. While considerable success has been found with all these methods of treatment, none is completely successful in all cases. Again, there is considerable need for 'individualizing' treatment for each woman and the state of her disease.

Several gynaecologists have noted that when the VIN is diagnosed in pregnant women they have seen spontaneous regression to normal skin when the baby has been delivered. In such cases waiting before offering treatment seems reasonable. The influence of pregnancy again calls into question the role of the immune system in this disease process, because in pregnancy the immune system may not function in the same way as it does normally. In the pregnant woman the immune system may be impaired, possibly to protect the baby from rejection as a 'foreign body'. It has also been reported that VIN has occurred in women with impaired immunity associated with other conditions such as leukaemia (cancer of the blood cells) and other cancers of the female reproductive organs.

Follow-up

As with CIN, women who have been treated for VIN and VAIN need extremely careful follow-up – usually with colposcopy examinations. They are especially at risk of developing new areas of abnormality and/or recurrence of already treated disease. Women who have had CIN treated will also need careful surveillance of their vaginas and vulvas. In a 1986 report of 59 women with VAIN, whose ages ranged from 23 to 72 years, half of them had already been treated for CIN and 71 per cent of them had more than one area of abnormality. Stage III abnormalities of the vagina (VAIN III) are, however, far less common than CIN III, and in a 1974 survey in America the incidence of VAIN III was 0.2 cases per 100,000 women compared to 36.4 cases of CIN III per 100,000 women. A decade later these figures have risen but the ratio remains about the same. Despite the relative rarity of both VIN and VAIN, those involved with screening for CIN will be on the lookout for signs of abnormalities developing in the skin of vagina, vulva and around the anus.

One particularly worrying fact to come out of a 1986 report on VAIN from Toronto in Canada was that 68 per cent of the women had previously undergone a hysterectomy: 48 per cent for the treatment of CIN or invasive cervical cancer, 10 per cent as part of the treatment for another gynaecological cancer and 42 per cent for non-cancerous problems such as heavy periods. This raises the question of whether women who have had a hysterectomy for non-cancerous reasons, and therefore do not need cervical smears, should be seen regularly thereafter to have a cytological check of their vagina and an inspection of the vulva. Certainly women who have had hysterectomies for CIN or cervical cancer ought to be considered for screening for VIN and VAIN.

9 The emotional impact

No one can overestimate the worry, fear and occasional panic that you may experience if you are told that your cervical smear report is anything but normal. Having been sensible by coming forward for a simple screening test, you are not prepared emotionally for the shock of being told that something, however trivial, is not satisfactory. It is this subconscious fear that prevents many women from requesting cervical and breast screening as often as they should – and, indeed, it also prevents men from requesting regular blood pressure measurement and other checks.

National screening programmes which personally invite every individual woman to come forward for screening are successful. The invitation in her hand helps a woman overcome the natural reluctance to enquire if there is anything wrong.

Hearing the news

Women are told of their smear reports in a variety of ways. One of the best is for you to receive a letter stating that the test was negative and advising you to have a repeat smear after a stipulated time interval – this serves as a reminder to plan the next smear. Many GPs and family planning clinics are moving towards this system.

Unfortunately many women are told that they will hear nothing if it is negative and only receive a letter if it is positive. This system causes a great deal of anxious waiting and occasionally leads to mistakes if letters are not sent or go astray. Some units say, 'Telephone the receptionist for the result in about two months.' Inevitably when you telephone there is a delay while the report is located and the result if it is not normal, and/or the instructions for when it should be repeated, may not be given clearly. Every system other than a clear, straightforward letter can cause anxiety.

Clearing up the confusion
It is not the responsibility of a doctor's secretary, or a GP's receptionist, or a Family Planning Clinic Organizer, to counsel women with abnormal smears. If you are confused, upset or surprised by your smear result, or have been asked to attend for repeat after repeat for months and months, you should take it up with the doctor or nurse who actually took the smears. The implications of the result and plans for the future can then be made, and the doctor or nurse can go through with you the possible reasons for the need for repeat smears quietly and in confidence. You can then be sure whether you need a repeat smear after a certain length of time or need to be referred for colposcopy.

Repeat smears
As can be seen from Chapter 2 there is a large number of reasons why the smear needs to be repeated earlier than usual. This often causes a great deal of worry and if this has happened on several occasions you can ask for a colposcopic examination anyway to ensure that all is well and, if necessary, to obtain treatment which will quickly return your smear result to unequivocally normal. This also takes the pressure from the cytologist in the laboratory, who may be anxious about the smear and requests frequent repeats to be safe. A quick colposcopy examination will sort this situation out.

The colposcopy visit

Like a visit to the dentist, waiting for the colposcopy appointment is a nerve-wracking experience. Although, like the dental visit, only good can come out of it, apprehension rather than relief is often experienced. The first shock you may have to face is the arrangement for the colposcopy appointment, as the waiting time may be two or three months or even more in some centres. This unhappy state of affairs leads to worries that the condition of the cervix will deteriorate while waiting; this is a fear also shared by doctors in colposcopy clinics. It will only be relieved when District Health Authorities provide adequate colposcopy facilities to ensure that women can be seen within a week or two of receiving the smear report. These women may well have waited two or even three months already for the result of their smear test and by now are getting to the end of their tether. It is difficult to be more than sympathetic about this situation at present, although much could be gained by concerted campaigns to improve facilities. However at least you know that once you are seen at the colposcopy clinic, treatment will be arranged quickly and is likely to be a hundred per cent effective.

Frustrations at the colposcopy clinic

Almost without exception colposcopy clinics in the UK are extremely busy, in an effort to see as many women as possible and to keep waiting times within reason and safety. The doctors and nurses in colposcopy clinics are usually working flat out from the beginning of the session to the end. But delays can occur in these clinics all too frequently. First of all many of the doctors who work in colposcopy clinics are busy gynaecologists and obstetricians – they will occasionally be delayed or called away by emergencies, although they usually make every effort to keep their colposcopy sessions sacrosanct. They will be bleeped, telephoned, Air-Called and Radiopaged during their colposcopy clinics – all of which will cause delay.

It is also very difficult to keep clinics running correctly to their appointment times. Some women will take five minutes to counsel and examine, some will take fifteen and a few half an hour. I have some patients who say 'Just get on with it and tell me what treatment I need and then get on with that', and some will ask me twenty or so questions before the colposcopy examination has even begun. Nobody wants to hurry a woman with such questions or skimp on counselling time if it is needed even if this inevitably delays the rest of the clinic.

Even in the best of clinics notes and/or smears and/or biopsy results are not immediately available when you arrive at the colposcopy clinic. Very occasionally this means you must wait until these are located or the relevant laboratory is telephoned to get the results dictated.

It is not difficult to understand why someone who arrives for a 10 am colposcopy appointment (after waiting two months for it) is fairly uptight if she gets in to see a doctor (who has been delivering a baby at 10 am) at 11 am or 11.30 am.

Taking it all in

Much of the time sitting down with the doctor in the colposcopy clinic before the colposcopy examination is spent asking questions. Date of the last period? Result of the smear before this one? Current contraception? History of vulval warts? Partner with penile warts? It may be that you are up on the colposcopy couch before you have had a chance to ask the doctor all the vital questions you had planned. Your mind may go a total blank as soon as you sit down in front of the doctor. Usually you may ask one or two questions which are particularly bothering you and then be fairly keen to get the colposcopy examination over with. Despite being given ample opportunity to ask questions afterwards it may not be until you have just left the clinic that more questions will suddenly come to you. By that time the busy doctor in the busy clinic will be examining another woman.

Some women write down their questions clearly at

home before they go for the colposcopy appointment and I have known several women who tape-recorded our pre-treatment conversation so that they could go over what we had discussed with their partners at home. Some doctors, however, may not welcome either approach, and subtle reference to your notes may be advisable! As medical students we are taught to be wary of the patient with a little list of symptoms or questions – 'maladie du petit papier' – and some doctors bristle at the thought of being tape-recorded. Not all, though; some use a video camera and screen to show a woman her own cervix and the areas of abnormality and they welcome interesting questions from their patients.

Short of a huge list of questions on several sheets of foolscap, it is often worthwhile having a few written notes (especially a record of the first day of the last menstrual period) to take into the doctor and to make a brief note of what the doctor has said and advised during the consultation. Of course, many doctors in colposcopy clinics write to their patients after the visit confirming what has been found and the treatment arrangements. And the colposcopy clinic nurse will reiterate what the doctor has said and occasionally give written instructions. I understand Claire Rayner was a general clinic sister who started writing down what her busy doctors had told patients so that the patients, who may have been flustered when with the doctor, could read her notes calmly at home. And so began her advice column.

Colposcopy – the inelegant position

Whereas most women dislike the thought of climbing up on to a colposcopy examination couch and splaying their legs into the foot supports, in practice this produces only a little anxiety at the time. The skill of the colposcopist and his or her nurse is to relax you and 'de-fuse' the situation. This is most often successful and you will find yourself on the couch chatting away happily about the weather, holidays, your job, your children, and so on, during the examination. Women usually consider that the implication of the disease and their desire to be treated far outweigh any initial anxiety about the examination itself, and often the examination surprises and pleases women by its brevity and reasonable comfort. If an experienced colposcopist cannot see, for example, the transformation zone upper limit in a woman with a smear indicating severe dysplasia, a cone biopsy will be selected and the size and extent worked out quickly with staining. This may only take a few minutes. By contrast, however, a relatively inexperienced colposcopist with a difficult cervix to evaluate may take up to 20 minutes and need several biopsies. Similarly if teaching is also undertaken the time you are up on the couch may be prolonged.

Treatment times can also vary greatly – from a 20 second application of the cold coagulator to a laser cone biopsy under local anaesthesia which may take half an hour. This sort of thing is of course very difficult to predict – every case is different and has to be treated accordingly.

Pain

Discomfort and actual pain can occur during the taking of the microbiopsies and during some forms of treatment. The woman who is relaxed and comfortable during the colposcopic examination and who has been well counselled about what to expect often finds the taking of one or a few biopsies produces no more than a light nipping sensation and very often no pain at all. A few, often nervous, women get very keyed up during the application of the acetic acid and iodine solutions, and the taking of the biopsy is the trigger to release their pent-up anxiety, often inducing faintness. Some distraction may be necessary such as talking to the clinic nurse or doctor, or deep breathing during the procedure which is causing most apprehension. A similar situation occurs during treatment procedures. It is a source of pride for the colposcopist when the woman cheerfully hops off the couch after her examination and/or treatment and announces, 'That wasn't too bad.' Thankfully this often the case.

After the treatment

Many women regard the whole experience with relief when it is all over. There is sufficient publicity around nowadays to worry any woman who is sexually active of the chance of developing an abnormality of the cervix. They are relieved when it has been caught in time and dealt with. The fear of a recurrence is ever present and most women resolve to keep their annual smear appointments after treatment without fail.

Some women I have talked to, however, regard the experience with resentment – not so much about the treatment as such but because, by needing it at all, they feel 'picked on'. In their self analysis they feel that they are no more culpable than many other women and cannot understand why they should be chosen to suffer. This is usually combined with the concept that 'a man has given me this'. Often they try to pinpoint which sexual encounter may have been responsible or in extreme cases have turned, perhaps unfairly, on their current partner and accused him of infidelity.

Some women regard the process of having a smear and subsequent colposcopy examination as an invasion of their body territory – an invasion which may leave them feeling vilified and unclean. It comes as a great shock to many young to middle aged women, perhaps those who would be included in the professional groups, including the 'young upwardly mobile', who have had only two or three sexual partners over ten or fifteen years and who have attended family planning clincs conscientiously to avoid an unwanted pregnancy, who have volunteered for regular cervical screening and then suddenly find themselves in the world of the colposcopy unit feeling hurt and degraded, especially if this is sited in a venereal disease clinic. Similarly this does not seem a fair 'reward' for being a conscientious and responsible citizen. But the only reward available in a cervical screening programme is a negative smear or the chance of early treatment for a positive one, and in the end the chance of avoiding a life-threatening disease has to over-ride all other considerations. There is not enough firm evidence of specific causes at the moment to enable any doctor to say categorically why abnormal cells occur, and it is not helpful to apportion 'blame' (see Chapter 7). All we can be sure of is that it *is* a sexually transmitted disease, which means that men are implicated, and need to be made aware of the fact.

As the concept of the male factor and the 'high risk' man gains more currency, with greater attention placed upon the sexual habits of the male partner, attitudes may change towards cervical cancer being a problem for both men and women. The present emphasis on 'safe sex' to avoid the spread of AIDS is equally applied to cervical cancer.

10 The case for screening

Cervical smear screening of the adult female population offers an opportunity to detect at the pre-invasive stage most of those women who will go on to develop invasive life threatening cervical cancer. When the women at risk have been identified they can then be investigated with colposcopy and appropriate treatment can be arranged which will prevent the development of the invasive cancer. Furthermore, those women can be carefully watched thereafter for any future signs of pre-invasive cervical cancer.

Two thousand women die of cervical cancer in Britain each year – many are mothers of young teenage children – and two-thirds of them have never had a cervical smear. Many of those who die are young themselves or in early middle age. Whereas the cure rates for invasive cancer are relatively high as compared to many other cancers, such as cancer of the lung caused through smoking, treatment of the invasive disease – surgery, radiotherapy, chemotherapy – involves considerable discomfort for the women who undergo the treatment, and they would be much better off if the disease had been detected and treated in the pre-invasive stage.

Success of screening

Following George Papanicolaou's announcements in the

1940s, women with gynaecological problems attending doctors were given a routine cervical smear, and by the 1950s screening had been offered to women without specific problems. Such was the enthusiasm for screening that no proper trials were conducted to see if it could be scientifically shown to be an effective means of preventing cervical cancer in the population as a whole.

By the 1960s many countries in Europe, including the United Kingdom, were practising 'well woman' screening. Opinion was divided for and against. Those funding what little screening was offered, mainly in the National Health Service and local authority clinics, were not sure if even the small sums spent on screening were cost-effective.

In the absence of large-scale trials (which would most likely be unethical in that they would involve having a group of women who were *not* screened for comparison) a good indicator of whether cervical screening is effective is to look at those countries where it has been practised in an organized way. In many smaller countries with a relatively low population of adult women at risk, screening has reached a high proportion of relevant women. In bigger countries, such as the United Kingdom, with larger populations, screening has reached a much smaller proportion of the female population.

It was reported in 1982 that in Iceland, Sweden, Finland and Denmark the age-adjusted incidence of cervical cancer increased until the mid-1960s and then fell sharply. In Finland, Sweden and Iceland country-wide screening was introduced at that time and was associated with this sharp fall in cervical cancer rates. In those three countries women were personally invited to participate in the screening programme. In Denmark there was a fall in the number of new cases of cervical cancer each year after 1965 but it was not such a steep decline; there was considerable local variation there in the way screening was carried out and only 40 per cent of women were personally invited.

In Norway no screening of women without symptoms was organized on a country-wide basis and there the rates of cervical cancer have continued to increase.

In Iceland groups of women up to the age of 50 were offered screening and in each group the incidence of cervical cancer fell. Older women were not initially included in the screening system and the fall in cervical cancer rates was not as marked as in the younger groups.

Cervical screening was introduced in Sweden in 1960 and it has been estimated that without a screening programme cervical cancer would by now have risen to the second or third most common form of cancer in that country, instead of being the fourteenth.

The British experience

In the United Kingdom the number of new cases of cervical cancer each year is still rising and it is doing so against the background of a sharper rise in the incidence of CIN, which many doctors feel has reached epidemic proportions. According to the Department of Health and Social Security, in 1975 2,498,000 cervical smears were taken in England and Wales, of which 11,911 were positive. In 1985, of 3,897,000 cervical smears, 35,752 were positive, which means that the proportion of positive smears had increased by over 50 per cent during this decade.

In Britain, there are about six million women under the age of 35 at risk from cervical cancer, and about twelve million at risk over that age. Yet only about four million smears are taken every year, and there is no way of knowing how many of those smears are repeats on the same person, perhaps because of cytology reports which have nothing to do with CIN in any form. Fifty-five per cent of those four million smears are taken on women under 35 and most are taken by general practitioners, who, as has already been noted, do not get any payment when offering this service to this age group.

In the past five years there has been a tiny drop – about one-twentieth – in the death rate in the under-35 age group, but most experts see the statistics showing this trend being reversed soon. It is probable that this slight drop in mortality is more to do with women coming forward earlier with the symptoms of an existing tumour, which is then cured (see Chapter 6), than because more women are having regular smear tests. And there has been no change in the death rate among women over 35 years of age.

It is thought that the number of cervical cancer cases each year would have risen more steeply without the screening services currently in operation. But until 70 per cent or more of women are screened regularly for cervical abnormalities there will not be a significant reduction in mortality. Screening hospital patients with gynaecological conditions is useful but leaves many women unscreened. In one north-west London hospital, 2296 women were screened, of whom 41.9 per cent had never had a smear before. Seventy per cent were over 39 years of age. Dyskariosis was found in the smears from 46 women and two women with negative smears had endometrial cancer (cancer of the womb lining). Thus 48 women screened had significant findings, giving a rate of 21 per 1,000. Eleven patients had CIN III – 4.8 per 1,000.

In many ways it seems extraordinary that Britain does not have a national screening plan. There is after all a *National* Health Service, in which a national maternity service operates quite efficiently. Instead funding is channelled through the regions to use as they wish, and cervical cancer screening has to fight its corner against other strong contenders for money such as heart surgery, kidney dialysis, neonatal intensive care and even breast cancer screening, something that cervical screening should be linked with, not competing against (see later).

Yet cervical screening is definititely cost effective. It costs the National Health Service between £2 and £5 to take a smear, depending on where it is taken. General practitioners are by far the cheapest source of smears in this context since they generally have lower overheads, and it is of course cheaper if the smear is 'tagged on' to a consultation with a woman about some completely different problem. Having the smear examined in the cytology laboratory and a report done is more expensive, because more skilled – the cost here is between £10 and £20 depending on the area. This has to set against the cost to the Health Service of treating a woman with full-blown cervical cancer, which can run into thousands of pounds if it requires radical surgery and expensive radiotherapy. This expenditure could be saved in almost every case and the resources channelled into other areas with a national screening programme to pick up and cure all women with cervical abnormalities before they become invasive.

A recent report from the British Medical Association (the doctors' trade union) described the present screening programme of hospital antenatal and gynaecological clinics, general practitioners and family planning clinics as uncoordinated and sporadic. There are few organized call and recall systems in Britain at the moment, although excellent systems have been introduced in some places such as Tayside and Aberdeen. However, the BMA report did draw attention to the lack of overall planning, with the Department of Health unable to supply the BMA with figures on the percentage of women screened, or on the number of them who later develop cancer. The report proposes greater communication between health authorities, family practitioner committees (who employ the general practitioners), laboratory cytology services and general practitioners. Local screening programmes and laboratory facilities are financed by the District Health Authorities, but it is the family practitioner committees who identify who is to be screened and who are responsible for call and recall.

The BMA report indicates that some family practitioner committees do not have a coordinated cervical screening policy, while others refuse or are unwilling to give the cytology laboratories information on their population index. Some District Health Authorities have been reluctant to apportion sufficient funds to their part in the system. Some family practitioner committees do not yet have a computer-organized call and recall system and those that have computers do not all have the same type of computer, which may prevent them from transferring smear records when women move from the area.

In 1986 the *British Medical Journal* reported the results of follow-up in Nottingham of women who had shown mild to moderate dyskariosis on their cervical smears. Those who had not been promptly followed up had a 29 per cent chance of harbouring CIN II, 22 per cent CIN III and an estimated 5 per cent having microinvasive or invasive cervical cancer. Of women with invasive cervical cancer another study reported that there had been a failure to follow up abnormalities in 15 per cent of them. The Nottingham study also reported on 50 women who had developed which in 43 was traced to failure of communication between the cytology laboratory, hospital clinics and general practitioners. Of significance in terms of the need for proper counselling, all of the seven who initially refused a further smear accepted the invitation when a full explanation was given.

Cytology laboratory facilities

Coincident with, and most likely related to, the publicity surrounding the death of a woman in 1985 in Oxford who had not been informed of an abnormal cervical smear, there has been a tremendous increase in the demand for cervical screening in the United Kingdom.

The Association of Scientific, Technical and Managerial Staffs (ASTMS) recently carried out surveys of the workloads of cytological laboratories and found them to be operating under very heavy pressure indeed. Almost all the laboratories in the surveys reported huge increases in the number of cervical smears being sent in with no similar increase in staff.

As mentioned in Chapter 2, the preparation and staining of the slides on which the cervical smear is sent to the laboratory can be partially automated but the slide must, at the moment, be scrutinized by trained personnel and abnormalities checked and reported on by consultant cytologists. Many laboratories also had problems with insufficient clerical staff who record, type out and send out reports. Salaries have been unattractive for the skilled cytology and clerical work involved, and many places remain unfilled. Many routine smears were waiting eight to twelve weeks for analysis – the best example in the surveys was two days and the worst was six months.

Breast cancer screening

Hard on the heels of appeals for an effective cervical screening programme have recently come calls for a national breast screening programme which, in some claims, would save the lives of up to 2,500 women a year. This raises the obvious possibility of providing a combined breast/cervix 'well woman' type of screening service. Currently some women are taught self breast examination by doctors and nurses with instructional leaflets available in doctors' surgeries and family planning clinics. Only about one in ten breast lumps is malignant and therefore a more accurate system of screening is necessary. By adding soft tissue X-ray screening (mammography), the accuracy of breast screening is improved greatly. Pick-put rates for breast cancer have been estimated from 3 to 5 per 1,000 women screened in general practice up to 23 per 1,000 in high-risk selected groups.

In Sweden a recent breast cancer screening project was found to have reduced the death rate in women with this disease aged 50 to 74 years by 40 per cent, detecting 70 per cent of cancerous lumps at the very earliest and potentially curable stage. Before the screening programme was introduced only 11 per cent were detected. The incidence of breast cancer in the more advanced stages was reduced from 80 per cent to 26 per cent. Because many of their cancers were detected in the early stage most women were treated with only the removal of a segment of breast tissue and not given post-operative radiotherapy.

The frequency of cervical smears

Recommendations for smear frequency have been changing over the last five years in a largely unsuccessful attempt to keep pace with the changing nature and development of cervical cancer and the steep rise in the incidence of CIN. There is general agreement that virgins do not need screening for cervical cancer. There is some evidence that genital wart virus (HPV) infections of the vulva and cervix can be transmitted in the absence of penetrative sexual intercourse, but for practical screening purposes cervical smears should only be taken once sexual intercourse has begun.

It is also generally agreed that if the first cervical smear is negative it should be repeated after one year to exclude a false negative result the first time. Many studies have shown that the technique of smear-taking may be inadequate in a substantial proportion of those taken because of failure to obtain an adequate and representative sample of all the cervical cells at risk. It is therefore necessary not to trust every first-time smear and to repeat it after a short interval at maximum of twelve months.

The present British screening policy aims to take cervical smears from all sexually active women every five years and early in pregnancy.

In a collaborative study reporting in 1986 of screening programmes in the USA, Canada and six European countries, it was found that relative protection was higher in women with two or more negative results of cervical smears than in those who had had only one negative smear, particularly in the first five years after the last test. There was little difference in the protection afforded by screening every year compared with every three years, but screening only once every five years offered significantly less protection. The other conclusion the study made was an obvious one – centrally organized screening programmes were more effective than uncoordinated screening.

The British Medical Association report referred to earlier recommended that women should be screened at three-yearly intervals. This followed a study which showed that reducing the interval from five to three years reduced the incidence of cervical cancer by 8 per cent. However, if smears were performed annually there would be a further 2 per cent drop.

How quickly can abnormalities develop?

As long ago as 1973 a survey showed that women with even low-grade CIN were 20 times more likely to develop CIN III than the general population and seven times more likely to develop invasive cancers of the cervix. By now these figures considerably underestimate the problem. Studies at the Middlesex Hospital in London in 1983 showed that the time interval between the first evidence of abnormal cells (CIN) and the development of CIN III was less than two years in over 80 per cent of patients. Two out of the three patients who developed invasive cervical cancer had negative smears two to four years before. Clearly, a shorter screening interval will prevent more cancers but at a progressively rising cost per cancer prevented.

The recommended five-year interval in Britain has been suggested as the cause of the relative failure to reduce the level of cervical cancers occuring each year as much as in other countries. Dr D.M. Parkin and colleagues reporting in the *British Journal of Obstetrics and Gynaecology* in 1985 estimated that the effect of screening about three million women and treating some 3,000 cases of CIN III each year in Britain is that the incidence of invasive cancers has fallen by only 23–37 per cent. This is a much smaller reduction than that estimated as possible by Dr E.G. Knox in the *British Journal of Cancer* in 1976, who predicted that a 77 per cent fall would follow five-yearly screening of women over the age of 35 years.

It has often been recommended that selective and frequent screening, say annually, for high-risk groups of women may be more cost effective. The argument against this is that many of those women most at risk are unlikely to book appointments for screening on their own initiative, and this explains why the countries with measurably successful programmes are those which have screened a very high proportion of the population by sending out personal invitations. In particular these systems include older women who would not normally be screened at the antenatal clinics, sexually transmitted diseases clinics and family planning clinics.

Safety first

There is a balance to be drawn between the need to screen and the screening facilities available at the moment or in the immediate future. It is essential that women make maximum use of what facilities exist to ensure those at greatest risk have reasonable access to accurate cervical smear taking and speedy cytological reporting. There must be adequate colposcopy facilities to investigate abnormal smears and adequate facilities for the treatment of CIN by laser vapourization, cold coagulation, cryocauterization, etc, and adequate operating time and facilities in hospitals to perform the necessary cone biopsies generated.

A working system

It would seem that from the knowledge of this disease we have at the moment and the patterns of change it is undergoing, cervical screening should be conducted by sending personal invitations to all women aged twenty to at least 55 to 60 years, to attend for a cervical smear. Those who fail to take up the offer should be further invited with a complete explanation of how the cervical smear may help them. With our current facilities smears should be repeated at least every three years. All patients with vulval or vaginal warts, or dyskariosis, on their cervical smear reports should be examined with a colposcope by an experienced colposcopist for further investigation and treatment. Women with inflammatory changes or mildly atypical cells on their cervical smear should have a repeat smear in three months' time, and if things are not back to normal by then, they should be referred for colposcopy. Considerable efforts must be made to ensure that smear results are communicated to both the women themselves and their general practitioners. An adequate computer-controlled call and recall system should exist with careful checks of follow-up systems, preferably with facilities to exchange information with computer-controlled systems in other areas of the country.

An ideal system

For the individual woman a preferred system would be an annual cervical smear, combined with a breast cancer screening system probably involving mammography in the higher age groups. Each woman would be sent reminders each year and there would be a thorough system for communicating results to women and their general practitioners. Cervical smears and breast screening results would be reported within one week. Later on it may be possible to include a screening system for cancer of the ovaries, such as by blood tests for tumour 'markers' and/or ultrasound examination of the ovaries.

The 'here and now'

However, in the absence of such an ideal system, women have to face the realities of the situation. In most cases, the onus is on you to find the facilities to be tested and then to follow up the result. A regular cervical smear does give protection against a cancer which currently kills over two thousand women a year in England and Wales. Go for it.

Helpful Organizations

Advice and counselling

The Health Education Authority
78 New Oxford Street, London WC1A 1AH (01–631 0930)

The Family Planning Association
27–35 Mortimer Street, London WIN 7RJ (01–636 7866)

The Patients' Association
Room 33, 18 Charing Cross Road, London WC2 (01–240 0671)

The Women's National Cancer Control Campaign
1 South Audley Street, London W1Y 5DQ
Founded in 1965 to help women overcome their fears about cancer and to take simple precautions which could well save their lives.

BACUP (British Association of Cancer United Patients)
121/123 Charterhouse Street, London EC1M 6AA (01–608 1661)

The Marie Curie Foundation
28, Belgrave Square, London SW1X 8BG (01–235 3325)
Offers counselling for patients and their families.

The Herpes Association
39 North Road, London N6

Brook Advisory Centres
233 Tottenham Court Road, London W1 (01–323 1522 or 01–580 2991)
Specialise in counselling younger women.

Independent health screening centres

Marie Stopes House
The Well Woman Centre, 108 Whitfield Street, London W1 (01–388 0662/2585)

PPP Female Health Screening
99 New Cavendish Street, London W1M 7FQ (01–637 8941)

BUPA Women's Unit
300 Grays Inn Road, London WC1 (01–837 6484)

Medical Express
Chapel Place, Oxford Street, London W1 (01–499 1991)

Index

Acetic acid solution 42
acquired immune deficiency syndrome 93
actinomycetes 30
age factor 103
AIDS *see* acquired immune deficiency syndrome
anteversion 10
anxiety 107–9
Ayre, J. Ernest 21

Biopsy 45, 48
blood vessels 41
brachytherapy 86
breast cancer screening 121
British Medical Association 119

Caesium 137 87
carcinogen 14, 91
carcinoma in situ 35
CAT *see* computerized axial tomography
cautery 15, 60–63
cervical intraepithelial neoplasia 49
cervicitis 26
chemotherapy 89
childbearing 97–8
CIN grading system 49–51
circumcision 92
clinics 17–19, 37–9
coil *see* intra-uterine contraceptive
cold coagulator 59–60
colposcope 36
computerized axial tomography 83
cone biopsy 65–73
cost effectiveness 118
cryocautery 57–9
Cusco, Edward 20
cystoscopy 83
cytology 22, 25, 120

Delays
  at clinic 109
  in laboratories 120
development rate 123
diaphragm 10
diathermia 60–63
dysplasia 33–4, 99

Ectropian 15
endometrial cells 14
erosion, cervical 15
EUA *see* examination under anaesthesia
examination
  couch 39, 111
  under anaesthesia 83
external radiotherapy 86–7

Fears 106–9
frequency of tests 121–2

Gardnerella 28
general practitioner 18, 117
gonorrhoea 29

Herpes genitalis 30
histopathology 85
HIV *see* human immunodeficiency virus
HPV *see* human papilloma virus
human immunodeficiency virus 93
papilloma virus 30–31, 94–6
hysterectomy 73, 84

Incompetent cervix 72–3
infections 26–31
inflammatory smear 26
insurance policies 63
internal radiotherapy 87
intra-uterine contraceptive 10, 30

intravenous urogram 82
invasive tumours 78–9
iodine solution 44
IUD *see* intra-uterine contraceptive
IVU *see* intravenous urogram

Koilocytosis 30, 33, 49

Laboratories 25, 120
laser treatment 53–7, 75
LAT *see* local ablative therapy
local ablative therapy 44
lymph nodes 79, 81–2

McDonald's stitch 72
male factor 91–2, 114
menstrual period 38, 53, 71
microinvasion 77
mortality rate 117
mosaicism 42
mucus, cervical 10

Nabothian follicles 16
National Health Service 118
NMR *see* nuclear magnetic resonance
nuclear magnetic resonance 83

Oral contraceptive pills 98
os 12
ovulation 10

Pain 112
Papanicolaou, George Nicolaus 6
pregnancy 38, 72, 105–6
proctoscopy 83
prognosis 89
progression rate 100–101
promiscuity 98–9
punctation 42

Questions 38–9, 110–111

Radical hysterectomy 84
radiotherapy 86–8
rectal intraepithelial neoplasia 95
repeat smears 31, 108
retroversion 10
RIN *see* rectal intraepithelial neoplasia

Saline washing 40
screening 19, 115–126
semen 92
sexual intercourse 56, 91, 96

smoking 96–7
spatula 21
speculum 20
squamous cells 12
staging 79

Telephone enquiries 31–2
teletherapy 86
thrush, 15, 27
transformation zone 14
Trichomonas 28
TZ *see* transformation zone

Upper limit 43
uterus 10

Vaginal intraepithelial neoplasia 95, 104
VAIN *see* vaginal intraepithelial neoplasia
venereal disease 29
villi 42
VIN *see* vulval intraepithelial neoplasia
virus infections 92–6
vulva 47
Vulval intraepithelial neoplasia 95, 104

Warts 30, 46, 94
womb *see* uterus